Advanced ECG

Advanced ECG:
Boards and Beyond

What You Really Need to Know
About Electrocardiography

Brendan P. Phibbs, M.D.
Professor of Clinical Medicine, Section of Cardiology,
University of Arizona College of Medicine
Chief of Cardiology, Kino Community Hospital
Tucson, Arizona

Little, Brown and Company
Boston   New York   Toronto   London

Copyright © 1997 by Little, Brown and Company (Inc.)

First Edition

Library of Congress Cataloging-in-Publication Data

Phibbs, Brendan P.
   Advanced ECG : boards and beyond : what you really need to know about electrocardiography / Brendan P. Phibbs.
      p.   cm.
   Includes index.
   ISBN 0-316-70512-8
   1. Electrocardiography.   I. Title.
   [DNLM: 1. Electrocardiography.   WG 140 P543a 1996]
RC883.5.E5P48   1996
616.1'207547 — dc20
DNLM/DLC
for Library of Congress   96-18845
                                                                CIP

Printed in the United States of America

MV-NY

Editorial: Tammerly J. Booth
Production Services: Textbook Writers Associates, Inc.
Indexer: Joan Croce
Production Supervisor: Louis C. Bruno Jr.
Designer: Marne Goodrich
Cover Designer: Sally Bergman-Costello

To the memory of Terese Kelly, a dark-haired, sparkling, courageous lady from Laughrea, County Galway (my mother, who died much too early when I was much too young)

Contents

Preface   ix

1. Sinus Rhythms: Two Benign Variations   1
2. Ectopic Beats and Sustained Ectopic Rhythms: Mechanisms of Idiorhythms and Paroxysmal Tachycardia   4
3. Differential Diagnosis of Wide-Beat Tachycardia   17
4. The Supraventricular Tachycardias   31
5. Various Abnormalities of Intraventricular Conduction   43
6. More About Aberrancy   61
Self-Assessment I   71

7. AV Block: Where Is It Localized and What Do You Do About It?   86
8. Diagnosis of Complex Forms of AV Block: Some Tricks, Some Booby Traps   110
9. Atrial Fibrillation   125
10. Atrial Flutter   138
Self-Assessment II   151

11. Preexcitation   162
12. Fascicular Beats and Fascicular Tachycardia   176
13. Concealed Conduction, Exit Block, Bundle-Branch Wenckebach, and Supernormal Conduction   183
14. Fatal Arrhythmias: Ventricular Fibrillation, Ventricular Flutter, Torsade, R-on-T Phenomenon, Standstill   191
15. The Sick Sinus Syndrome   198
16. Digitalis-Toxic Arrhythmias   206
17. Myocardial Infarction   218
18. Diagnosing Myocardial Infarction in the Presence of Bundle-Branch Block   254
19. Transient Myocardial Ischemia and Angina Pectoris   267
20. Pericarditis   273
21. Enlargement of the Chambers of the Heart: Hypertrophy and Dilatation   278

22. "Nonspecific" Myocardial Pathology   291
23. Electrolytes and Drugs   303
24. Two Special Cases: Pulmonary Emboli and Hypothermia   310
Self-Assessment III   313

25. Graduation Exercise   335
26. How to Take a Board Examination   348

Appendixes

 I. Indications for Pacing in the Bradyarrhythmias   363
II. How to Determine Axis   368

Index   373

Preface

If you're a physician who trained in the United States, you were cheated. You've been neglected. You're entitled to a sense of outrage.

Electrocardiography is a basic life-and-death skill that's going to confront you with harrowing decisions throughout your professional life, but chances are that all through your residency and fellowship training you never had any organized formal training in it. Your instructors thought you were going to learn electrocardiography by osmosis or by ionic exchange or by breathing the air of the university hospital.

How do I know this? I know it because I served several terms on the ECG Interpretation Committee of the ACC and because, on my own, I surveyed teaching hospitals across the country from Boston to San Francisco. *Eighty percent of teaching hospitals have no organized ECG-arrhythmia training in residency or fellowship programs.*

Whenever I lecture to residents and fellows I hear the same complaint: "Why don't we get more of this stuff? We really need to know it!"

Okay chaps,* you're right. You certainly do need to know this stuff. That's what *Advanced ECG: Boards and Beyond* is for. It's based on the tutorial sessions I lead with the fellows in our program at the Veteran's Hospital in Tucson.

This book isn't going to waste your time with baby steps: it's assumed you know how the leads are hooked up and what a P wave is. This is a book for you to use when you're ready to start functioning in the real world as a clinician. In fact, the first arrhythmia illustrated in the book is one I guarantee you'll run into as a question on the Internal Medicine Boards.

In your clinical life you're not going to start with simple cases and go on to complex ones: your very first night in the emergency room or in the coronary care unit may bring you face to face with some incredibly

---

*"Chaps" is a unisex term.

complex *gemisch* of wide and narrow beats, anomalies of AV conduction, and variations of aberrancy, and you'd better be able to dissect the ECGs and react intelligently. I think I can honestly say this text will help you do just that. I say so on the basis of responses from students, residents, and fellows I've trained over the years using exactly the methods and many of the figures in this book.

The language in *Advanced ECG: Boards and Beyond* is deliberately simple. Don't be surprised when you read that "the fast AV nodal channel likes to conduct backward" instead of "the fast AV nodal channel exhibits preferential retrograde conduction." The two statements are in fact identical, and the simple language is chosen with considerable care. This book is written to be as different as possible from the gibberish that came with your computer!

Electrocardiography is an elegant, basically simple, totally logical means of diagnosis that gives more pragmatic information that any other diagnostic mode in cardiology.

Learn it!

Good hunting!

B. P. P.

Advanced ECG

1 | Sinus Rhythms: Two Benign Variations

Wandering Pacemaker

This is a completely harmless, totally insignificant variation of a sinus rhythm. The shape of the P wave changes from beat to beat, but the timing of the beats doesn't. The rhythm is regular and uninterrupted even though the P waves look different. Sometimes the contour of the P wave will change from upright to inverted and then back to upright (Fig. 1-1A and B). You distinguish this from ectopic firing by a simple observation. There are no premature beats. The rhythm doesn't change. All that changes is the shape of the P waves.

This phenomenon is important only because it is sometimes confused with significant arrhythmias (one text even refers to it as a form of sick sinus syndrome!).

The peculiar change in P wave shape is a result of "wandering" of the sinus impulse in the region around the sinoatrial node. The deeply inverted P waves suggest that the pacing site has "wandered" toward the upper reaches of the AV node — a region often described as the "coronary" node.

FIGURE 1-1A and B
Two examples of wandering pacemaker. In each strip the P wave changes its shape from upright to inverted and back again *with no change in rhythm.* This consistent rhythm is important because it distinguishes the innocuous wandering pacemaker from true ectopic firing.

A

B

I have seen cardiologists confuse this harmless phenomenon with multifocal atrial tachycardia, a really significant arrhythmia. This is inexcusable! In multifocal atrial tachycardia there are showers and runs of premature beats from many different sites in the atria (more about this later). With a wandering pacemaker — to say it one more time — the rhythm is *regular;* all that changes is the shape of the P waves.

Change in Sinus P Wave Morphology with Rate

When the rate increases, the sinus P waves will sometimes "peak," assuming a taller, steeper shape. When it slows, they resume their more rounded shape (Fig. 1-2). This is another sinus variant of absolutely no significance: Don't confuse it with ectopic atrial rhythms.

Sinus Arrhythmia

Take your pulse; now take a deep breath in and then exhale. Your pulse rate probably slowed when you exhaled. This is the normal type of variation in sinus node discharge associated with the breathing cycle (Fig. 1-3). It may be quite exaggerated, especially in the young, but it's harmless.

The clinically significant disturbances of sinus node function will be described in Chap. 15, The Sick Sinus Syndrome.

FIGURE 1-2
Strip from an event recorder with sinus rate varying from 59 on the left to 110 on the right. Note the striking increase in amplitude of P waves. (The loss in R wave amplitude was not rate-related but was simply due to a change in body position when the patient turned on the recorder.)

FIGURE 1-3
Sinus arrhythmia. Sometimes respiratory variations in rhythm can be quite striking, as in this strip, but they're harmless. There are rare forms of sinus arrhythmia that are independent of the breathing cycle.

2 | Ectopic Beats and Sustained Ectopic Rhythms: Mechanisms of Idiorhythms and Paroxysmal Tachycardia

If you're an internist or a cardiologist, sooner or later you're going to find yourself taking an ECG competency test. It may come as part of the Internal Medicine Boards or the Cardiovascular Boards, the ACC Competency Test, or a hospital ECG privileges examination. In every case you can be certain you'll confront a problem like the one shown in Fig. 2-1. Is the right answer obvious? Read on!

When you study ectopic beats and sustained ectopic rhythms you have to acquire two sets of skills. First you have to be able to decide where the ectopic focus lies anatomically. Is it atrial, junctional, or ventricular? Most of the time this is a simple diagnosis, but it can get tricky.

Second, you have to decide what kind of ectopic firing is going on. Ectopic beats and ectopic rhythms will always be the result of one of two mechanisms: reentrant or automatic. It's critical to decide which mechanism is at work, because treatment and prognosis are completely different; fortunately, it's usually easy to make the distinction.

Determining the Source of Ectopic Beats

You probably already know how to localize ectopic beats, but here are some fine points.

FIGURE 2-1
A patient has suffered an inferior wall MI. Eighteen hours later the rhythm illustrated here appears. The blood pressure is 130/80, the patient is pain-free, and all vital signs are normal. Choose one of the following treatments.
1. lidocaine
2. isoproteronol
3. atropine
4. pacemaker
5. no treatment

Atrial Ectopic Beats

You need to remember three facts. First, if a beat arises in an atrial ectopic focus, it will generate a P wave with a different shape from the sinus P wave. This difference in shape may be slight or extreme, but it will always be detectable (Fig. 2-2).

Second, the P-R interval of the atrial ectopic beat will always be 0.12 seconds or more, never less. It will usually be longer than the P-R interval of the sinus beats. In other words, the track from sinus node to AV node is the most efficient track from atria to ventricles. If a beat arises somewhere else in the atria, it will usually take longer than the sinus beat to reach and traverse the AV node.

Third, a beat arising at any given site in the atria will produce a characteristic P wave specific for that site. This is important in the diagnosis of multifocal atrial tachycardias (Fig. 2-3).

These are small points, but they may be important in analyzing complex arrhythmias.

FIGURE 2-2
Premature atrial beats from a number of foci. Note the difference in P wave morphology — sometimes striking, sometimes minimal, but always different from the sinus P waves.

FIGURE 2-3
Multifocal atrial rhythm. This is when P wave morphology becomes critical. You can identify at least four different atrial foci from the shape of the ectopic P waves.

Junctional Beats

Most beats arising in the junction will be conducted *forward* (antegrade) into the ventricles and *backward* (retrograde) across the atria. As a result there will be some combination of a normal narrow QRS with a retrograde P. The retrograde P may come just before, during, or after the QRS (Fig. 2-4). The relation of the atrial and ventricular complexes depends on the speed of conduction *back* across the atria compared to the speed of conduction *forward* across the ventricles.

If the retrograde impulse excites the atria before the antegrade impulse excites the ventricles, the P wave will come just ahead of the QRS. The P-R interval will always be less than 0.12 seconds. When you see a fixed short P-R interval (less than 0.12 seconds), you're looking at junctional beats (Fig. 2-4A).

FIGURE 2-4
Junctional rhythms. The retrograde P wave may come (A) just before, (B) during, or (C) just after the junctional QRS.

A

B

C

At this point you interrupt: "Wait a minute! What about preexcitation? That will certainly produce a fixed short P-R." Good question. The difference is that the P wave of the junctional beat will have a "retrograde" morphology — completely different from the shape of the sinus P waves. It will usually be inverted in the inferior leads. With preexcitation you see normal sinus P waves with a short P-R.

If the retrograde impulse excites the atria at the same instant that the antegrade impulse excites the ventricles, you won't see the P wave because it will be hidden in the QRS. Thus a narrow QRS not preceded by a P wave must be junctional (Fig. 2-4B). If the retrograde impulse reaches the atria after the antegrade impulse reaches the ventricles, the retrograde P wave will follow the QRS (Fig. 2-4C).

Odd and unexplained fact: In theory, the QRS of a junctional beat should look exactly like the QRS of the sinus beat; after all, both impulses come down the same ventricular track. However, sometimes the QRS of a junctional beat will be quite different from the QRS of the sinus beat. Nobody is quite sure why this happens, although it may be that the junctional beat breaks out into the bundle branch system from an eccentric point of entry. The practical point is that even though the shape of the QRS is different, the beats are still junctional (Fig. 2-5).

Ventricular Ectopic Beats

The bizarre QRST and the absence of a preceding P wave are obvious and need no further discussion. However, there is one critical difference between junctional and ventricular ectopic beats; learn this difference now and it will help you on many dark nights in the emergency room when you're looking at a wide-beat tachycardia. During a junctional tachycardia the junctional beats are practically always conducted retrogradely across the atria. This retrograde impulse discharges the sinus node before it can fire. The ventricles and the atria are activated from the

FIGURE 2-5
There are a number of junctional beats on this strip. Most of them have a different contour from this sinus QRS. All the beats after the first beat are junctional with a QRS that is taller and different in composition from the sinus beats. (There's no S wave in the junctional beats.) Sometimes the difference is more striking than this.

same source: the junction. In contrast, about half of all ventricular ectopic beats, whether single or occurring during a tachycardia, are not conducted back up through the AV node. The sinus node is *not* affected and goes on firing independently. The atria and ventricles are dissociated for one beat, the atria responding to the sinus node and the ventricles to the ectopic beat. In Fig. 2-6 you can see the sinus P wave inscribed near the end of the T of the VPC.

Since the sinus impulse marches undisturbed right through the VPC, and the next sinus beat comes in right on time, you will see a "full compensatory pause" — that is, a pause that is exactly double the sinus interval. Remember, about half of all VPCs are dissociated from the sinus rhythm, so when you see dissociated P waves during a wide-beat tachycardia, the diagnosis is *ventricular* tachycardia. Keep this simple observation in mind; you'll use it later in this chapter.

The other half of all VPCs are conducted retrogradely across the atria, just like the junctional beats, except that the atrial impulse always follows the QRS (Fig. 2-7).

If an ectopic beat arises out in the distal subendocardium of the ventricle, it will always be at least 0.12 seconds wide in the adult heart — sometimes more, but never less. This is a surprisingly consistent finding. (Formerly there was a lot of speculation about "narrow" VPCs; it turns out that these are really "fascicular" beats, arising in the fascicles of the bundle branch system, hence the more rapid propagation. Fascicular VPCs and fascicular tachycardias are covered later in this chapter.)

FIGURE 2-6
Ventricular ectopic contraction with a dissociated sinus P wave. As a result the interval from the P ahead of the VPC to the one after it is an exact double interval, or full compensatory pause.

FIGURE 2-7
Ventricular ectopic beats with retrograde P waves.

Determining the Mechanism of Ectopic Beats

Reentry

Pick up any strip in your CCU with a lot of VPCs on it and look at it carefully (Fig. 2-8). Note that the VPCs come at a precisely fixed interval after the sinus beat. The ectopic beats are "linked" to the preceding sinus beat with an exact, unchanging coupling interval. You'll find this kind of linkage about 98% of the time, whether the ectopic beats are atrial, junctional, or ventricular.

Any mathematician will tell you that when you see that kind of precise association more than five or six times, it cannot possibly be a coincidence. There has to be a *causal connection* between the sinus beat and the ectopic beat. Somehow the passage of the sinus impulse "triggers" the ectopic beat.

We now know how that happens: it's called "reentry" (Fig. 2-9). To set up reentry, there must be an area of one-way block somewhere in the Purkinje fibers (Fig. 2-9A). (One-way block is fairly common; you'll see an obvious example of it later in this chapter.) There must also be an area of very slow conduction (Fig. 2-9B). Because of the one-way block, the outgoing activating impulse isn't conducted forward normally in one small area. As a result this area of conducting tissue remains unactivated, still ready for stimulation. In most parts of the chamber the normal activating impulse moves swiftly, at 4 m/sec. However, there's that slowly conducting area mentioned above; it's moving so slowly that it "reenters" and activates the blocked part of the system *after* the rest of the chamber has recovered and is ready to conduct again. This reentrant impulse breaks out into the chamber and produces the ectopic beat. Thus the ectopic beat is in fact caused by the passage of the sinus impulse — that's why the two beats are linked. It's as if the sinus impulse flipped a little pinwheel that went through one rotation and fired at a fixed interval after the sinus beat. You'll see this constant linkage whether the reentrant ectopic beats are atrial, junctional, or ventricular.

Reentry may produce single ectopic beats; on the other hand the reentry circuit may produce paroxysmal tachycardia when it goes on firing

FIGURE 2-8
Reentrant ventricular ectopic beats. Note the precisely fixed interval to the preceding sinus beats.

FIGURE 2-9
Diagram of reentry.

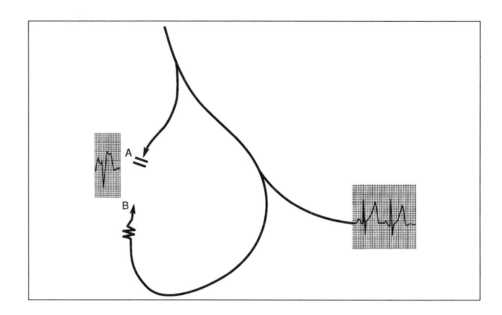

FIGURE 2-10
Paroxysmal ventricular
tachycardia, a reentrant
rhythm.

rapidly and regularly. Reentrant ectopic beating is always abnormal and sometimes dangerous (Fig. 2-10).

Automatic Ectopic Beats

Far back in the evolution of life, God or somebody saw to it that the heart had a "fail-safe" system. If the sinus node fails (and it can), there has to be some other means of generating a heartbeat or the species will die off very quickly.

Fortunately there are hundreds of "reserve" pacemakers scattered through the heart, chiefly in the AV node and junction and in the ventricles. These are small areas of tissue in the subendocardium that can fire as pacemakers (Fig. 2-11). They can build up a potential and discharge just the way the cells in the sinus node do. They may discharge one beat or they may go on firing, producing a sustained ectopic rhythm. These sustained ectopic rhythms are the "idio" rhythms: idiojunctional or idioventricular. They practically always fire in the slow to high-normal range.

There are several kinds of automatic rhythms. It's important to distinguish between them since they have very different clinical implications.

FIGURE 2-11
An automatic ectopic focus. At A the passage of the normal sinus impulse has suppressed the ectopic focus. At B something has halted the normal activating impulse; after a certain fixed period the automatic focus is "released" to begin discharging, setting the rhythm of the heart.

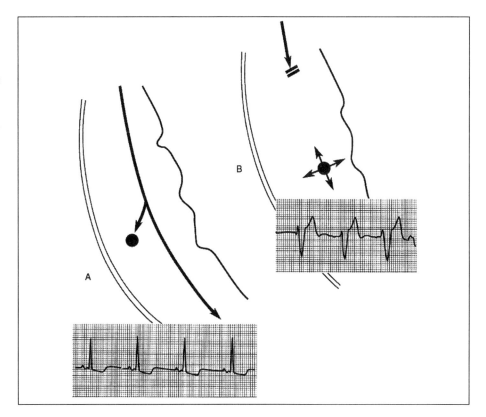

AUTOMATIC-DEMAND. This is the way an automatic focus is supposed to function. It fires only when the heart rate falls below a certain critical number, exactly like an implanted demand pacemaker. The ectopic focus "waits" for a certain preset interval before it fires: If a normal impulse doesn't come along during that period the ectopic rhythm takes over.

Automatic ectopic foci are suppressed by the passage of the normal activating impulse. To use an intern's phrase, the passage of the normal activating impulse keeps the automatic ectopic pacemakers "pounded down." When the normal impulse fails, the ectopic focus is said to "escape" from the dominance of the sinus impulse. The length of time that must pass before the ectopic focus can fire is called the "escape interval" of the ectopic pacemaker.

FIGURE 2-12

(A) Idiojunctional rhythm, rate 50. There is no sign of atrial activity, so it's clear that failure of the sinus node is the reason for the appearance of the idiorhythm. Perhaps it's a sick sinus?

(B) Idioventricular rhythm. Note the retrograde P waves. The ectopic focus is discharging the atria by retrograde conduction, thus suppressing sinus node activity.

(C) A sinus pause followed by an idiojunctional rhythm, rate about 30. The sinus pause was caused by retching, a powerful vagal stimulant. Here the idiojunctional rhythm is essential to maintain hemodynamics.

To reiterate, these automatic foci fire only when the normal impulse fails. They're often lifesaving.

Automatic rhythms may be idiojunctional or idioventricular (Fig. 2-12 A, B, and C). (One of many errors you'll find in some texts is the statement that idioventricular rhythms are inherently slower than idiojunctional rhythms. In fact the two types of rhythm overlap in rate and there's no definitive difference.)

When a slow idiorhythm appears, of course, you have to ask what's wrong with the normal mechanism. Heart block? Sick sinus? Look for the cause whenever you see an idiorhythm.

ACCELERATED AUTOMATIC-DEMAND: ACCELERATED IDIORHYTHMS. For reasons that are not clear, these automatic-demand pacemakers may become overactive; that is, they may fire when they're not really needed. Imagine an overenthusiastic lifeguard who comes dashing out to rescue you when you're only knee-deep and don't need rescuing. Or imagine a thermostat that's set too high so that the furnace keeps turning on when the house is already warm enough. To be more exact, imagine a demand pacemaker that's set to fire whenever the heart rate drops below 80. The problem with these accelerated-demand pacemakers is that they don't wait long enough before they start firing — their "escape interval" is too short. The normal pause after a premature beat or a slight slowing of the sinus rhythm is often all it takes to release one of these automatic foci. The accelerated idiorhythm begins firing and often takes over the rhythm of the heart for some time (Fig. 2-13A and B).

Accelerated idiorhythms may perform a useful function. If there's failure of normal conduction, such as AV block, the "escape" rhythm that takes over may fire in the "accelerated" mode — that is, in the range 55–110. When you see an accelerated idiorhythm, always look for the cause. Was there some serious failure of the normal rhythm that let the idiorhythm escape? Or is the idiorhythm simply an example of an "overexcited" ectopic focus getting in the way of a perfectly adequate normal rhythm? Either way, in the vast majority of cases these accelerated idiorhythms are harmless — if not actually helpful — and require no treatment.

Now go back to Fig. 2-1 and mark the right answer — it's "no treatment," of course. You'd be surprised to learn how many candidates get that specific question wrong every year!

FIGURE 2-13
(A) Accelerated idiojunctional rhythm. There are occasional sinus beats competing with an idiojunctional focus firing at a rate of 75. Note that as soon as there is a slight pause in the sinus rhythm the junctional focus "escapes" and takes over. It's not serving any useful purpose, but it's probably not hurting anything.

(B) The first five beats are sinus beats. Then there's a sinus pause, and the junctional focus escapes and begins discharging at a rate of 65, just fast enough to "get in the way" of the sinus impulses. The sinus node recaptures the rhythm in the last two beats. Harmless, no treatment needed.

Very rarely, a sustained accelerated idiorhythm can cause problems in a hemodynamically compromised patient because of loss of atrial "kick." In those cases the answer is to get rid of the slight pauses that are the cause, by eradicating the premature beats or speeding the sinus rate by drugs or pacing. This is rarely necessary.

AUTOMATIC TACHYCARDIAS. Rarely, an automatic focus may fire in the paroxysmal tachycardia range, 130 or higher. Automatic tachycardias may arise in the atria, the junction, or the ventricles. These are relatively rare arrhythmias with special characteristics; they will be described in a later chapter.

AUTOMATIC-PARASYSTOLIC. The other type of automatic firing is parasystolic. A parasystolic focus is a tiny area of tissue somewhere in the subendocardium that behaves like a totally independent pacemaker. It fires at its own rate and breaks out to produce a beat whenever it happens to hit the right instant between beats — when the tissues are out of their refractory period and receptive to stimulation.

The curious thing about parasystolic foci is that there's an area of "protection block," or one-way block, around them so that they aren't affected by the passage of the normal activating impulse (Fig. 2-14). The parasystolic focus is a little anarchist that bangs away at its own independent rate and captures the rhythm of the heart whenever it gets a chance.

Parasystolic beats differ from reentrant beats and automatic-demand beats in that they have no connection whatsoever with the preceding si-

FIGURE 2-14
Parasystole. A parasystolic focus is illustrated at A. It fires away at its own rate with no relation to the normal heart cycle. At B the protection block around the parasystolic pacemaker is illustrated. The normal activating wave can't get in to discharge the ectopic focus, but the focus can and does get out whenever the surrounding tissues are out of their refractory period.

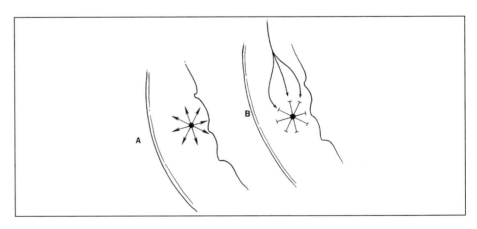

nus beat. The interval from the sinus beat to the ectopic beat varies wildly (Fig. 2-15). This is one of the markers of parasystolic firing.

There's another way you can recognize parasystole: Since the parasystolic focus goes on firing at its own rhythm, the beats will always appear at an interval that's a multiple of the basic rate of the focus. In other words, you can reduce the interval between parasystolic beats to a least common denominator that represents the basic rate of the focus.

Parasystolic rhythms are rare. They have no particular function, though they may serve a useful purpose if they happen to be firing when the normal mechanism fails — but it's accidental when they do.

To summarize, ectopic beating may be the result of one of the following mechanisms.

1. Reentrant: Always abnormal and sometimes dangerous. Paroxysmal tachycardia is usually caused by sustained reentry.

2. Automatic-demand: A physiologic and often lifesaving response, idiojunctional or idioventricular, exactly like a demand pacemaker. Rate slow to low-normal, 40–60.

3. Accelerated automatic-demand: accelerated idiorhythms: An automatic focus that fires in the normal to high-normal range. Usually they're not needed; they're like demand pacemakers that are set too high, so that they interrupt a perfectly normal heart mechanism. Rate low to high-normal, 60–110.

FIGURE 2-15
Ventricular parasystole. The ventricular ectopic beats have no fixed relation to the preceding sinus beats, and they appear at their own regular rhythm.

4. Automatic tachycardia: A rare phenomenon with special clinical features, occurs when an automatic focus in the atria, junction, or ventricles fires in the tachycardia range, 130 or higher.

5. Automatic-parasystolic: An independent automatic rhythm, unaffected by the normal activation of the heart. No consistent linkage to conducted beats; parasystolic beats appear at intervals that are multiples of the basic rate of the parasystolic focus. Locus may be atrial, junctional, or ventricular. Parasystolic rhythms may serve a useful purpose if one happens to be discharging when the normal mechanism fails, but it's an accident when they do. Rate low to high-normal, 40–110.

3 | Differential Diagnosis of Wide-Beat Tachycardia

It's 2 A.M. in the emergency room and you confront an ECG like the one shown in Fig. 3-1. You see a rapid succession of wide QRS complexes without obvious P waves, rate 180. Your mental computer flashes two possible diagnoses:

1. Ventricular tachycardia.
2. Junctional tachycardia with bundle-branch block.

Prognosis and treatment are at opposite poles; the distinction may well be of life-and-death importance.

You need some basic tools, some specific ECG skills, to tackle this problem. You must be able to recognize the following:

Bundle-branch block
Rate-dependent bundle-branch block
AV dissociation
Capture beats
Fusion

FIGURE 3-1
Wide-beat tachycardia. Is it ventricular or junctional with bundle-branch block? You couldn't possibly make a diagnosis from this strip alone.

Bundle-Branch Block

This is a topic that is often made needlessly complex. In theory and practice, it's simple: V1 is the defining lead in bundle-branch block. The logic consists of three elements:

1. If a supraventricular beat produces a QRS that is 0.12 seconds or more in width, one bundle branch must be blocked.
2. If V1 consists of a wide S wave, left bundle-branch block is present (Fig. 3-2).
3. If V1 consists mainly of a wide terminal R wave, right bundle-branch block is present (Fig. 3-3A, B, and C).

As you can see, right bundle-branch block V1 may consist of a small r followed by a wide, tall R (rR'), a plain R wave, or a qR. The essential point is that the last two-thirds of the complex consists of a wide R wave. In simple terms, the wide R wave is over the blocked ventricle. There will of course be a corresponding wide S wave over the normally activated bundle-branch area.

(Some descriptions of this topic are fantastically complicated with vectors and mean emf and interfaces, but you can safely ignore all this. Look at V1, apply the simple differentiation above, and you're on solid ground.)

FIGURE 3-2
Left bundle-branch block is defined by a wide S wave in V1; duration of total complex, 0.12 seconds or greater.

V1-V2-V3

FIGURE 3-3
Variations of right bundle-branch block patterns in V1. At A there's the classic rR', at B there's a simple R wave, and at C there's a qR because the patient has had an anterior myocardial infarct. The wide terminal R is the defining phenomenon for right bundle-branch block.

V1-V2-V3

A

V1-V2-V3

B

V1-V2-V3

C

Rate-Dependent Bundle-Branch Block

This is the simplest form of transient aberrancy. (Remember, the word "aberrant" means "deviating from normal form or pathway." Bundle-branch block is the extreme form of ventricular aberrancy.) Rate-dependent bundle-branch block means that one bundle branch has a prolonged refractory period; that is, it takes longer than normal for it to recover from each transmission. If the next impulse comes along before

FIGURE 3-4
(A) Abrupt slowing of rate from 62 to 43: The bundle-branch block disappears. It resumes when the rate goes to 68 for one beat and then disappears when the rate falls to 54. (B) Rate-dependent bundle-branch block.

the "tired" bundle branch has time to recover, it can't transmit, and the ECG will record bundle-branch block.

Figure 3-4A and B illustrate rate-dependent bundle-branch block. In Fig. 3-4A the difference in rate is substantial, but in Fig. 3-4B the first three beats are normally conducted at a rate of 73 (whereas bundle-branch block appears at a rate of 75). As you can see, the difference in rate between normal conduction and rate-dependent bundle-branch block may be very slight. In Fig. 3-4 there is normal conduction at a rate of 75 and bundle-branch block at a rate of 78.

Curious phenomenon: Figure 3-5 was recorded during treadmill testing. In Fig. 3-5A you see normal conduction at a rate of 90. The patient went into rate-dependent left bundle-branch block at a rate of 100, and the test was stopped. In Fig. 3-5B you see the pattern of left bundle-branch block *still present at a rate of 90.* For some reason it often requires a slower rate to come out of bundle-branch block and back to normal conduction than it did to go into bundle-branch block in the first place.

In Fig. 3-6 there's a typical example of rate-dependent bundle-branch block coming and going with slight variations in sinus rate; aberrancy also disappears with the pause after a ventricular ectopic beat. There is normal conduction in the beats marked "N" at a rate of 65. The first aberrant beat (A) in the top strip comes at an R-R interval equivalent to a rate of 75. In the bottom strip aberrant conduction persists at a rate of 71. When you're puzzling over wide beats and narrow beats you must be ready to recognize "critical" rate-dependent aberrancy, which comes and goes with very small differences in rates.

From all this comes a first step in logic when you're looking at an intermittent wide-beat tachycardia. When you see wide QRS complexes at a rapid rate and normal ones at a slower rate, you can consider rate-dependent aberrancy. On the other hand, when you see wide QRS complexes at a slower rate than the narrow ones, forget about rate-dependent aberrancy. The wide beats must be ventricular (Fig. 3-7).

FIGURE 3-5
Paradoxical persistence of rate-dependent bundle-branch block.

FIGURE 3-6
Rate-dependent bundle-branch block. The beats labeled "A" are aberrant; the beats labeled "N" are normally conducted. Note the very small difference in rate that sets up the aberrancy.

Dissociation

In Chap. 2 we discussed the phenomenon of atrio-ventricular dissociation. Dissociation means that the atria are being driven by one pacemaker (usually the sinus node) while the ventricles are being driven by an ectopic rhythm in the junction or the ventricles. The two rhythms are

FIGURE 3-7
Strips recorded a few minutes apart on the same patient. The wide beats in the top strip appear at a rate of 140. The narrow beats in the bottom strip appear at a rate of 150. You can't attribute the wide beats in the top strip to rate-dependent aberrancy: They must be ventricular.

independent. This is a critical observation in the diagnosis of wide-beat tachycardia because about 50% of the time ventricular tachycardia will be dissociated from an independent sinus rhythm. There are discernible independent P waves "marching through" the ventricular complexes.

With rare exceptions, junctional tachycardia is not dissociated. The ectopic focus lies at the edge of the atria, so the impulse is conducted back across the atria discharging the sinus node.

Here's a one-way correlation: If you see a dissociated sinus rhythm during a wide-beat tachycardia, the tachycardia is ventricular (accuracy about 98%). On the other hand, if you don't see dissociation, the tachycardia could still be ventricular. About 50% of all ventricular tachycardias will not be dissociated.

Sometimes the dissociated P waves are obvious, sometimes not. In Fig. 3-8 the P waves are sharp and well defined with a double "spike." You can put your calipers on them and march them through the wide-beat tachycardia; the unmistakable sharp deflection is obvious at the points marked "P."

It's not always that easy. Sometimes you have to turn to the Old Testament: "Doth the leopard change its spots?" Obviously not; the author of Isaiah was trying to make a point. Look at Fig. 3-9. There's a wide-beat tachycardia. The T waves keep changing their shape. Leopards don't change their spots and T waves don't change their shape. Further, the Q-T interval will be fixed at any given rate.

FIGURE 3-8
Dissociated sinus P waves "marching through" a short run of ventricular tachycardia.

FIGURE 3-9
Wide-beat tachycardia. Note the striking change in T wave morphology. Sometimes you can see well-defined peaks: These are obviously dissociated P waves. The tachycardia must be ventricular.

In Fig. 3-9 the T waves are changing their shape from beat to beat and the Q-T interval seems to be varying wildly. There's only one possible answer: AV dissociation is present, and the changing shape of the T waves means that there are dissociated P waves marching through them. Learn to look for changes in T wave morphology and Q-T interval in a wide-beat tachycardia. That's how you can spot dissociation and make a precise diagnosis.

Fusion Beats

When I talk to audiences of internists about arrhythmias I often ask if anyone would like me to review fusion. Invariably a great many hands go up.

Fusion beats are the 100% infallible marker for a ventricular source of wide beats. They are also called "Dressler beats" for the man who first described them. Figure 3-10A and B shows what happens.

To have a fusion beat you must have AV dissociation — the atria must be beating independently. In Fig. 3-10A you see a normal sinus impulse at A. This impulse has traversed the atria and is partway through the AV node when an ectopic ventricular focus fires at B. Now the ventricle is invaded by two impulses that meet, or "fuse," somewhere in the ventricular network. The result will be a beat like the one shown in Fig. 3-10B, labeled "C."

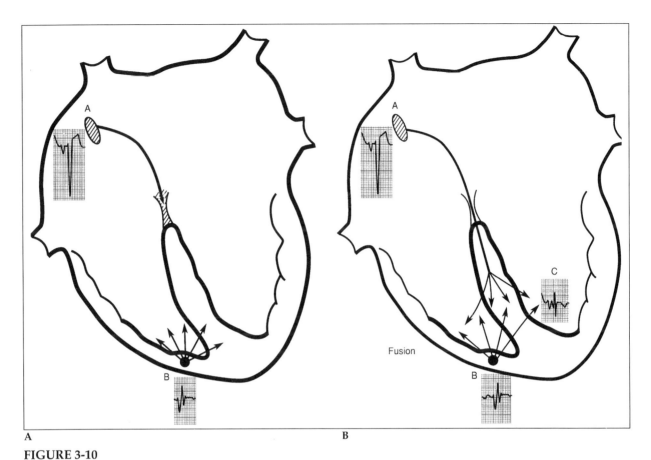

A   B

FIGURE 3-10
(A) Beginning of a fusion beat. (B) Fusion beat. The sinus impulse (A) and the ventricular ectopic beat have "collided" or fused in the ventricles, producing a hybrid beat at C.

The QRS will be a hybrid, with a morphology that lies somewhere between the shape of the sinus QRS and the shape of the ventricular ectopic beat. Note that beat C has a general outline like the ectopic beat except that it's narrow. The ventricular ectopic beat has been "normalized" to some extent by the invading sinus impulse. For fusion to take place, the ventricular focus has to discharge while the sinus impulse is still in the AV node. Therefore the P-R interval will always be shorter than the P-R of normal sinus beats.

One more time: Fusion beats will be characterized by a short P-R compared to the sinus beats. The QRS will be intermediate in shape between the QRS of the sinus beats and the QRS of the ventricular ectopic focus.

The fusion beat may look like a slightly widened and distorted sinus beat or it may look like a slightly narrowed and "normalized" VPC. It all depends on which impulse penetrates farther into the ventricle. Figures 3-11, 3-12, 3-13, and 3-14 are all examples of fusion beats. Study them carefully. This is a basic skill you'll exercise in many tense moments in the coronary care unit.

FIGURE 3-11

The beats marked "N" are normal sinus beats. The beats marked with a question mark might be ventricular, or they might be junctional beats with aberrant conduction. The beat marked "F" is the answer. It has a shorter P-R and a QRS that's intermediate in shape between the sinus beats and the wide beats. Obviously it's a fusion beat, and the wide beats must be ventricular.

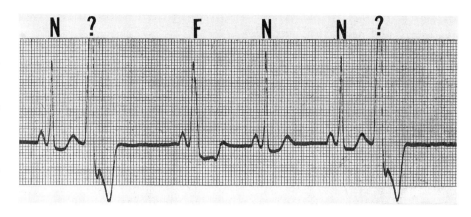

FIGURE 3-12

You saw this strip in the last chapter. It's reproduced here again because it's such a good example of a fusion beat. Obviously the beats marked with a question mark must be ventricular.

FIGURE 3-13

Normal sinus rhythm with occasional wide beats (V). At F there's an obvious fusion beat. The ninth and fourteenth beats are also fusion beats.

Capture

Fusion beats represent a partial capture of the rhythm by the sinus node. Sometimes the sinus impulse "sneaks through" between the beats of a ventricular tachycardia and penetrates the entire ventricular network, actually producing a normal sinus beat right in the midst of the ventric-

FIGURE 3-14
Sinus rhythm. At V, one obvious fusion beat.

FIGURE 3-15
Four-beat runs of ventricular tachycardia interrupting a sinus rhythm. You can see dissociated sinus P waves marching through the tachycardia with fusion beats (f) and a capture beat with a normal QRS. This strip illustrates all the criteria for the precise diagnosis of ventricular tachycardia.

ular arrhythmia. To have capture beats, of course, you must have a dissociated sinus rhythm.

When you see a capture beat, you use the logic you used to detect rate-dependent aberrancy: If you see a normal narrow QRS appearing at the same R-R interval as the wide beats, you have ruled out rate-dependent aberrancy as a cause of the wide-beat tachycardia. Logic!

The tracing in Fig. 3-15 illustrates all the criteria for the precise diagnosis of ventricular tachycardia. There are short runs of wide beats. If you look closely you can see dissociated sinus P waves marching through the wide-beat rhythms. The beat marked "c" is a capture beat. The QRS of the capture beat is normal even though it appears at the same R-R interval as the wide beats. The beats marked "f" are obvious fusion beats with a short P-R and an intermediate QRS morphology.

With all this information you can make a 100% infallible diagnosis of ventricular tachycardia. Try making the same observations in Fig. 3-16.

So far, this has been a one-way street. The criteria listed up till now are diagnostic of ventricular tachycardia. However, you won't find them in more than 50% of cases of ventricular tachycardia (some investigators put the percentage as low as 35–45%). If none of these criteria are present, it doesn't mean that you're not dealing with ventricular tachycardia. In at least half of all cases of ventricular tachycardia, the ectopic impulses are conducted back up through the AV node and across the

FIGURE 3-16
Ventricular tachycardia with dissociated sinus P waves, capture with fusion (c_f) and capture with normal QRS (c).

atria. There's no dissociation, so there's no chance for capture or fusion. How do we establish a diagnosis in these cases?

At this point I can predict the reader's question: "How about morphology? Can't you tell the difference between ventricular beating and aberrancy by the way the QRS looks? You certainly hear enough about it." Back in the sixties, Marriott launched an attempt to differentiate ventricular ectopic beats from aberrantly conducted supraventricular beats by the *shape* of the complexes. Over the intervening years many other investigators, including Wellens, Lie, Akhtar, Brugada, and Josephson have pursued this possibility.

There are indeed some characteristics of QRS morphology that enable you to say, with about 98% accuracy, that a given wide-beat tachycardia is in fact ventricular:

1. Wide QRS complexes: more than 0.15 seconds.
2. Uniform, totally positive or negative complexes across the precordium. No R/S complexes in the precordium.
3. Extreme axis (see Appendix II on axis measurement).
4. Deep S V6.
5. R/S complexes with a prolonged interval from R to bottom of S (more than 100 m/sec.).
6. Notching near the nadir of the S wave in V1 when V1 consists of a wide S.

Figures 3-17, 3-18, and 3-19 illustrate many of these features.

FIGURE 3-17
QRS morphology of ventricular tachycardia. The ventricular beats are about 0.16 seconds wide. (Note the frequent fusion beats.)

FIGURE 3-18
Ventricular tachycardia. The distance from the beginning of the R to the bottom of the S is 0.16 seconds (Brugada's sign of ventricular ectopic complexes).

FIGURE 3-19
Ventricular tachycardia, lead V1. Note the slurring just before the nadir of the S waves. This is evidence of ventricular tachycardia (Josephson's sign). Note that these beats look narrower than usual for ventricular tachycardia, but part of the QRS is "buried" in the baseline: They're really 0.12 seconds wide.

How about QRS morphology in aberrancy? There's an enormous and frustrating overlap between ventricular tachycardia and junctional tachycardia with aberrancy when it comes to QRS morphology. *If* none of the above characteristics are present, and *if* there is a three-component R wave in V1 (rsR') then there's a chance — no better than 80% — that the wide beats are caused by aberrancy. There are no specific characteristics of QRS morphology that permit you to say, with acceptable accuracy, that a given wide-beat tachycardia is in fact due to aberrancy — 80% simply isn't good enough for what may be a life-and-death decision. You can often very accurately rule ventricular tachycardia *in*, but you can't rule it *out*. This chapter is therefore going to conclude with an editorial.

The Aberrancy Aberrancy

Ventricular tachycardia is a dangerous arrhythmia: It practically always connotes significant organic heart disease. Conversely, junctional tachycardia with or without aberrancy is relatively benign. It frequently occurs in otherwise normal individuals. Because of the various studies trying to differentiate the two on the basis of QRS morphology, there's a dangerous and deplorable tendency for physicians in emergency departments and intensive care units to look at a wide-beat tachycardia, mutter that it "looks aberrant," and order potentially lethal treatment. Ventricular fibrillation, death, and malpractice suits are likely to follow in horrid swift succession.

Always apply these steps in logic:

1. Treatment for supraventricular tachycardias includes verapamil, digitalis, and phenylephrine. Any one of these is likely to be lethal if the tachycardia is really ventricular.

2. On the other hand, drugs used to treat ventricular tachycardia (lidocaine, procaine amide, and quinidine) will not do any harm if the rhythm is in fact junctional. Procaine amide or quinidine may well stop a junctional tachycardia.

3. There are many criteria, as listed above, that enable you to say that a given wide-beat tachycardia is in fact ventricular. These criteria are specific, but they're not sensitive. Many cases of ventricular tachycardia — possibly half — won't fit any of these criteria, so you're stuck with a diagnosis of "wide-beat tachycardia, possibly ventricular."

4. On the other side of the coin, there are no criteria that permit you to say with acceptable accuracy that a given wide-beat tachycardia is *not* ventricular and is in fact caused by aberrancy. In other words, it's a one-way correlation — a fact that often escapes many clinicians and investigators. (Many of my colleagues are brilliant observers but not very good logicians.)

There's only one sure way to diagnose aberrancy in this setting. *If* you find a previous tracing with sinus rhythm and bundle-branch block and *if* the contours of the wide-beat tachycardia are the same as the bundle-branch configuration when the patient was in sinus rhythm, then and only then can you diagnose aberrancy with confidence.

Here's a reasonable protocol for a wide-beat tachycardia:

First, always try vagal stimulation by carotid sinus massage, the diving reflex, or the Valsalva maneuver. If the tachycardia stops, you can be absolutely sure it was supraventricular.

Second, if vagal stimulation doesn't work, try adenosine. If this stops the tachycardia you can be sure it was supraventricular.

Third, if none of these maneuvers work, if there's no previous ECG for comparison, and if you value your patient's life, *treat for ventricular tachycardia!*

4 | The Supraventricular Tachycardias

There are six different, well-defined types of supraventricular tachycardia:

1. AV nodal reentrant tachycardia — the most common cause of paroxysmal supraventricular tachycardia.
2. AV nodal reciprocating tachycardia — the term *reciprocating* means that there's a bypass tract that forms a reentrant circuit with the AV node.
3. Automatic or "nonparoxysmal" junctional tachycardia.
4. Ectopic atrial tachycardia of childhood (relatively rare).
5. Sinus reentrant tachycardia — the rarest of the six.
6. Multifocal atrial tachycardia.

AV Nodal Reentrant Tachycardia or Two-Track AV Nodal Reentry

It's only in the last decade that we've learned what really happens in this very common arrhythmia. Figure 4-1 is a good illustration of the

FIGURE 4-1
Dual AV nodal pathways. In the top strip, the P-R interval is 0.20 seconds. In the strip immediately below, the P-R has abruptly lengthened to 0.48 seconds. These two intervals varied back and forth erratically even though the heart rate remained the same. There are obviously two separate pathways through the AV node, one fast and one slow.

underlying pathophysiology. (This isn't the best-preserved ECG in my collection — I had to rescue it from the wastebasket at our Veterans' Hospital, but it's such a rare and striking example of dual AV nodal pathways that it's reproduced here as well as possible.) You'll note that there are two different, well-defined P-R intervals, one prolonged (0.46 seconds) and one normal (0.20 seconds). These two P-R intervals appear erratically with no apparent reason for the change.

Tracings like this were the first evidence of *dual AV nodal pathways*. The only way you can possibly explain the random change in P-R intervals is that there are two completely separate AV nodal pathways that are isolated from each other. In other words, when an impulse comes down one pathway it doesn't affect the other. Invasive EP studies have shown that many individuals have dual AV nodal pathways, even though they don't show up in the surface ECG.

There's a slow pathway with a short refractory period, and a fast pathway with a long refractory period. Figure 4-2 shows what can happen. Normally conduction comes down the fast pathway, but sometimes a beat will be conducted down the slow pathway — usually this will be a premature atrial beat. Now there's the electric activity of the slow pathway still moving down the node when the fast pathway has fully recovered from its last transmission and is ready to conduct again. As one investigator put it, "the fast-track loves to conduct backward," or to state it in medical gobbledygook, "fast-track tissue manifests preferential retrograde conduction." Either way you say it, part of the impulse from the slow track enters the fast track and goes back up the AV node. Up at the

FIGURE 4-2
Mechanism of AV nodal reentrant tachycardia. In patients there is a "slow track" and a "fast track." Normally the activating impulse comes down the fast track (A). Sometimes the impulse comes down the slow track (B). Part of this impulse then enters the fast track and travels back up toward the atria while another part goes on to stimulate the ventricles. At the top of the AV node the returning impulse "bridges" very slightly into the atrial tissue and turns back down the slow track, thus perpetuating the cycle (C). Of course, the returning impulse also sends an impulse across the atria, producing a retrograde P wave. This is a typical "slow-fast" reentry; the cycle may also be reversed with a "fast-slow" track.

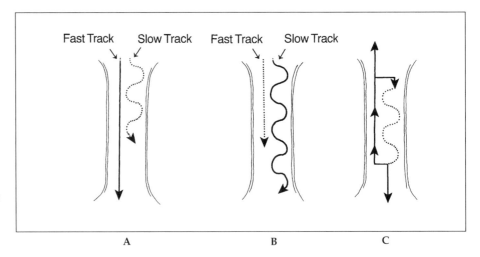

top of the AV, very slightly into the atrial tissue, the impulse reenters the slow pathway and starts back down.

Thus you have a reentry circuit right in the AV node. Of course, this reentry circuit throws off antegrade impulses that go on down into the ventricles and retrograde impulses that go back across the atria (Fig. 4-3). At other times the activating impulse may come down the fast track and back up the slow track. Thus, you may have either a "slow-fast" or a "fast-slow" reentry circuit in the AV node.

Note how this process starts in Fig. 4-3. The fifth beat is a premature atrial beat: Typically, this starts the reentry circuit. For the first few beats the retrograde P waves have changing relationships to the QRS complexes, depending on speed of conduction up and down. Toward the end of the strip the relation of retrograde P to QRS settles down and becomes fixed. This is typical of the beginning of one of these AV nodal reentrant tachycardias (AVNRT).

Figures 4-4, 4-5, and 4-6 are all examples of this type of arrhythmia. They constitute more than 90% of the supraventricular tachycardias you will see in the average emergency room or intensive care unit. The retrograde P waves may come just before, during, or after the QRS, depending on the relative speed of conduction back into the atria and forward into the ventricles. The rate will be rapid, in the range of 150–250.

Since this is a nodal rhythm, anything that depresses AV nodal conduction will turn off the reentry circuit and stop the tachycardia. Vagal stimulation, adenosine, digitalis, calcium blockers, beta blockers, and quinidine are all effective. It's logical to try vagal stimulation first by carotid sinus massage, the diving reflex, or the Valsalva maneuver. Adenosine is the next step: Between vagal stimulation and adenosine you can terminate more than 90% of these tachycardias. Remember, these interventions stop the arrhythmia abruptly and completely. If the

FIGURE 4-3
Diagram of typical AV nodal reentrant tachycardia.

FIGURE 4-4
AV nodal reentrant tachycardia, rate 214. Note retrograde P waves in bottom two leads.

FIGURE 4-5
Onset of AV nodal reentrant tachycardia. Note that a premature atrial beat triggers the tachycardia (beat no. 4, top strip). Note also that there's some variation in the relation of P to QRS in the top strip while the rhythm "builds up." In the bottom strip the relation of retrograde P to QRS becomes fixed.

FIGURE 4-6
Typical AV nodal reentrant
tachycardia, rate 187.

rate slows and then speeds again, you're not dealing with AVNRT. Look for another mechanism and another cause. AVNRT will almost always produce retrograde conduction across the atria. AV dissociation is very rare with AVNRT. AVNRT will never be the result of digitalis toxicity.

AV Nodal Reciprocating Tachycardia: "Preexcitation" Tachycardia

Figure 4-7 illustrates this simple mechanism. There's a bypass tract — some type of preexcitation. An impulse comes down the AV node and back up the bypass tract, forming a self-perpetuating circuit. It may also go around the other way, down the bypass tract and back up the AV node. (You'll read much more about this in the chapter on preexcitation, but it's introduced here to keep the record clear and complete.)

FIGURE 4-7
Diagram of AV reciprocating cycle involving a bypass tract. In this case the impulse comes down the AV node and goes back up the bypass tract. It can also go the other way.

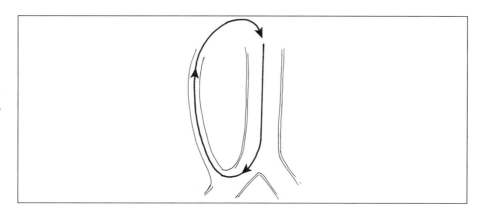

If the impulse comes down the bypass tract the QRS will often have the typical deformity of Wolf-Parkinson-White conduction, so the diagnosis is simple (Fig. 4-8). If, on the other hand, the impulse comes down the AV node, the QRS will be normal, and it's difficult to decide if there's a bypass tract. One clue may be helpful: The impulse returning to the atria, back up the bypass tract, will naturally arrive at the atria *after* the antegrade impulse reaches the ventricles, so the retrograde P will come after the QRS. That should at least arouse your suspicion of a bypass tract (Fig. 4-9).

The rate will be the same as in AVNRT: The arrhythmia will begin and end abruptly. In other words, this is a true paroxysmal tachycardia.

Since the AV node forms one arc of the circuit, anything that depresses AV nodal conduction can end the arrhythmia, just as with AVNRT. Vagal stimulation, adenosine, and suppressive drugs will all be effective. In addition, drugs that depress conduction in the bypass tract — e.g., procaine amide and quinidine — can end the arrhythmia.

Special note: You may have heard cautions about using AV nodal suppressant drugs like digitalis in the presence of preexcitation. That applies only when there's atrial fibrillation or flutter with a bypass tract. When the only arrhythmia is a simple paroxysmal tachycardia, you can

FIGURE 4-8
Reciprocating tachycardia with typical preexcitation deformity. The top two strips show intermittent WPW preexcitation with occasional normal beats. The second beat in the top strip is normal, with a P-R of 0.22 seconds and a narrow QRS. Most of the other beats on the top two strips show a much shorter P-R (0.13 seconds), with a very wide QRS — a typical WPW deformity. In the bottom strip there is a tachycardia in the same patient with a rate of 160 and the same wide QRS complexes, only modified a little by the rapid rate.

FIGURE 4-9
Reciprocating tachycardia with "orthodromic" conduction, meaning that the impulse comes down the AV node and back up through the bypass tract. The retrograde P *following* the QRS suggests that this is really a reciprocating tachycardia.

depress either side of the circuit and stop the arrhythmia. Response to treatment will be abrupt, all-or-nothing, just as with AVNRT.

This arrhythmia, like AVNRT, will practically never be dissociated: The retrograde impulse practically always discharges the sinus node. This arrhythmia occurs spontaneously: It is not a digitalis-toxic arrhythmia. A good abbreviation for this arrhythmia would be AVPET: AV Nodal Preexcitation Tachycardia. Nobody's proposed it yet, but it seems very reasonable, it's descriptive, and it's easy to pronounce. Why not?

Automatic or "Nonparoxysmal" Junctional Tachycardia

This is a simple type of arrhythmia; the only problem has been the inexcusably confused terminology.

Sometimes an automatic focus in the region of the AV junction begins to fire in the "accelerated" mode. The rate may be as low as 70 or as high as 130. You could properly call these either "accelerated junctional rhythm" or "automatic junctional tachycardia," depending on the rate (over or under 100). Instead they're all lumped under the term "automatic junctional tachycardia." How can you call something with a rate of 70 or 80 a "tachycardia"? Good question. The answer usually given is that you expect an automatic junctional rhythm to be slow, so a rate of 70 or more is a "relative" tachycardia!

The term *nonparoxysmal* is used because these arrhythmias don't have the abrupt, all-or-nothing beginning and end of the true paroxysmal tachycardias: They can begin and end more gradually.

Several features distinguish automatic junctional tachycardias from AVNRT and AVPET:

1. Automatic junctional tachycardias are often dissociated from the sinus rhythm (Fig. 4-10). It's common to see dissociated sinus P waves

FIGURE 4-10
Automatic junctional tachycardia dissociated from a sinus rhythm. The junctional tachycardia has a basic rate of 128. You can clearly see independent sinus P waves marching uninterrupted through the tachycardia. Every now and then you see a QRS appearing early, which tells you that the sinus node has "captured" a beat (for example, the second beat in the top strip: the sinus P wave is hidden in the preceding T). The sinus capture beats are labeled "S." This kind of dissociation is very rare with AVNRT or AVPET but is common with automatic junctional tachycardias — an important differential point!

FIGURE 4-11
Accelerated junctional rhythm, rate 88. This is also called an "automatic junctional tachycardia" even though the rate really isn't in the tachycardia range.

"marching through" the junctional rhythm and occasionally capturing a beat.

2. The rate of these arrhythmias is much slower than the rate of true paroxysmal tachycardias (Figs. 4-11 and 4-12).

3. Onset may be gradual, and there are often no symptoms.

4. Automatic junctional tachycardias are very commonly caused by digitalis toxicity. The only treatment required is removal of the offending drug.

FIGURE 4-12
Automatic junctional tachycardia, rate 102. The large "spiky" deflections that appear at the right-hand end of both strips are really dissociated sinus P waves: This patient happened to have massive atrial enlargement with bizarre P waves on the monitor, as recorded here. Again we see AV dissociation, common with this group of arrhythmias.

Ectopic Atrial Tachycardia of Childhood

This is relatively rare. It's caused by the discharge of an ectopic focus in the atria. The AV node is only a passive conductor in this arrhythmia — unlike AVNRT, it has nothing to do with the actual machinery. The actual mechanism may be a very small reentry circuit around an area in the atria or simply acceleration of an ectopic atrial focus.

The ECG is characterized by definite P waves with a consistent morphology, obviously different from the sinus P waves, and a P-R interval that is at least equal to the sinus P-R (Figs. 4-13, 4-14, and 4-15). The rate will usually range from 130 to 160 — somewhat slower than AVNRT or AVPET.

This arrhythmia commonly appears early in life and tends to persist into adulthood. Although it isn't dangerous, it can be seriously disabling. Sometimes it can be controlled with drugs, but invasive treatment with ablation is often necessary.

Sinus Node Reentrant Tachycardia

This is probably the rarest of the group. It's simple to picture: There's an abrupt increase in rate, but the P waves look exactly like the normal sinus P waves (Fig. 4-16). There appears to be a kind of micro-reentry circuit involving the sinus node that starts and stops abruptly, like any reentrant tachycardia. The rate will be somewhat slower than the AVNRT-AVPET group, in the range of 130–160.

Sinus node reentrant tachycardia starts and stops abruptly — that's how you distinguish it from a simple sinus tachycardia, which will always speed up and slow down gradually. Unless there's some coinci-

FIGURE 4-13
Ectopic atrial tachycardia. Note well-defined but bizarre P waves with normal P-R interval.

FIGURE 4-14
Short runs of ectopic atrial tachycardia. Note the striking difference in morphology between the sinus P waves and the P waves of the ectopic focus.

dental disease in the AV node, the P-R interval during the tachycardia will be identical to the sinus P-R.

This, too, is a "nuisance" tachycardia, usually responsive to suppressive drugs. As far as anybody knows, it is not caused by digitalis toxicity, but the literature on the subject is scanty.

Multifocal Atrial Tachycardia

This is a tachycardia with a single, specific cause.

On the electrocardiogram you see runs of atrial ectopic beats appearing in rapid succession with wildly differing P wave morphologies (Figs. 4-17 and 4-18). Remember that in Chap. 2 it was emphasized that each ectopic atrial focus produces a specific, characteristic P wave: When you

FIGURE 4-15
End of a run of ectopic atrial tachycardia. The relatively slow rate (128) and the obvious difference between the ectopic P waves and the sinus P waves are characteristic.

FIGURE 4-16
Sinus node reentrant tachycardia: abrupt onset and end, P waves and P-R interval identical to sinus impulses.

FIGURE 4-17
Multifocal atrial tachycardia (top strip). Resumption of sinus rhythm interrupted by random atrial ectopic beats from multiple foci in bottom strip after treatment with O₂ and magnesium.

see P waves with differing shapes it's obvious that a number of ectopic foci are discharging.

To diagnose multifocal atrial tachycardia (MAT), therefore, you must document rapid atrial ectopic beating from multiple foci. The diagnosis of MAT means that there are runs of three or more ectopic beats — single

FIGURE 4-18

Multifocal atrial tachycardia (top strip). Slowing of rate in bottom strip with multifocal single atrial, junctional, and ventricular ectopic beats, after treatment with O_2 and magnesium.

premature atrial beats, even though they come from multiple foci, are not the same thing. MAT practically always appears in short bursts of varying length as in Figs. 4-17 and 4-18. The result will usually be a completely irregular rhythm that could very easily be confused with atrial fibrillation. Look for the multiform P waves!

This is an hypoxic arrhythmia, and the treatment is proper oxygenation. Ordinary suppressive drugs like digitalis are not effective. In our institution we have been using intravenous magnesium, which has given encouraging results with control in over half of all cases. (This, of course, is still investigational.)

Paroxysmal Atrial Tachycardia with Block

This is an arrhythmia with a very specific clinical connotation. About 90% of the time it is the result of digitalis toxicity. It differs in many respects from the tachyarrhythmias listed here and will be described where it belongs: in Chap. 16, Digitalis-Toxic Arrhythmias.

5 | Various Abnormalities of Intraventricular Conduction

You're already familiar with simple bundle-branch block. There are other forms of intraventricular conduction delay; recognizing them is sometimes critical. Mastery of all the variations of intraventricular conduction is an absolute prerequisite for anyone claiming competence in ECG interpretation.

In this chapter you will learn how to recognize six distinct entities:

1. The normal septal Q wave. (The septal Q wave is important in some conduction defects; it's also a good idea to define it properly now so that you'll distinguish it from the pathologic Q waves of myocardial infarction.)
2. "Incomplete" bundle-branch block.
3. Intermittent bundle-branch block.
4. Normalizing fusion.
5. The hemiblocks, or fascicular blocks, and bifascicular and trifascicular blocks.
6. Nonspecific intraventricular conduction delay.

This may seem an intimidating list, but these are everyday workhorse skills. Normalizing fusion and intermittent bundle-branch block are not academic curiosities: They pop up in every busy emergency room and coronary care unit, and the electrocardiographer must be ready to recognize them.

The Septal Q Wave

When impulses pass from atria to ventricles, the left side of the septum is activated slightly before the right. Thus a small left-to-right force is generated (Fig. 5-1). This will be recorded as an initial negative deflection in any lead out to the left of the septum — avl, V5-6, or sometimes the inferior leads, II-III and avf. This Q wave will be *narrow* — it will never be more than 0.02 seconds wide in a normal heart.

FIGURE 5-1
Genesis of the physiologic septal Q wave. The activating wave moves through the septum from left to right, producing a small initial negative force in leads to the left of the septum.

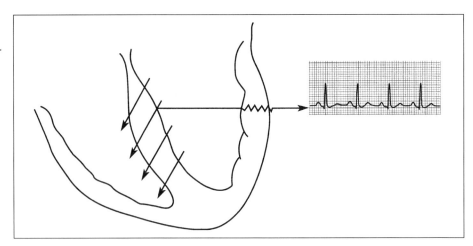

FIGURE 5-2
Septal Q waves in I and avl.

Sinus rhythm; Rate 102, PR 13, QRS 08, axis -30 left axis deviation otherwise within normal limits.

BRENDAN PHIBBS, MD 6/3/92im

Figures 5-2, 5-3, and 5-4 are all variations of the normal septal Q. Remember, it's the *width* of the Q that tells you whether it's physiologic (septal) or pathologic (necrotic). We used to emphasize depth of Q, but careful pathologic correlations have shown it's the *width* that's the crucial element. (I've seen some really tragic mistakes when normal septal Qs were misread as pathologic Q waves — hence the emphasis on this topic here.)

FIGURE 5-3
Septal Q waves in the inferior and anterior-lateral leads: II, III, avf, and V5-6.

FIGURE 5-4
Small septal Q waves in the sinus beats, not present in the VECs.

"Incomplete" Bundle-Branch Block

Sometimes you'll see an ECG that looks exactly like left or right bundle-branch block with one difference: The QRS is a little narrower than it is in true bundle-branch block — 0.10 or 0.11 seconds instead of 0.12 (Figs. 5-5 and 5-6). Nobody knows exactly what this means. My own ECG has shown a progression from "incomplete" right bundle-branch block with a QRS of 0.10 to "complete" right bundle-branch block with a QRS of 0.12 over the past eight years: The morphology remains precisely the same but the QRS is slightly wider.

I-II-III aVR-aVL-aVF V1-V2-V3 V4-V5-V6

Rhythm [II] 10mm/mV

FIGURE 5-5
"Incomplete" left bundle-branch block. The deflection is negative in V1, but the QRS is only 0.11 seconds wide and there's a septal Q in avl, indicating that there must be some conduction down the left side of the septum.

It has been postulated that in "incomplete" bundle-branch block the malfunctioning bundle is actually conducting slowly, while complete bundle-branch block means that it doesn't conduct at all. Nobody is sure, and the whole topic would be nothing more than an ECG curiosity except for one critical difference: A change from "incomplete" to "complete" bundle-branch block can be critical in the diagnosis of myocardial infarction.

Look at Figs. 5-7 and 5-8. Both have a left bundle-branch block configuration, but there are two important differences. First, the QRS complexes are narrower in Fig. 5-7. Second, there is a septal Q in avl in Fig. 5-7 but not in Fig. 5-8.

Think of the genesis of the septal Q as outlined above and take another look at Fig. 5-1. To have a septal Q the normal activating wave has to come down the left side of the septum *first* and penetrate the septum from left to right. If the left bundle branch is blocked, that can't happen. The activating impulse has to come down the right bundle branch, and the septum has to be activated from right to left. There cannot possibly be a septal Q wave.

Thus the classic diagnosis of left bundle-branch block must include the statement "no septal Q wave." Presumably, with the "incomplete" type of left bundle-branch block, there is penetration down the left side of the septum, albeit slow — hence the presence of the septal Q.

FIGURE 5-6
"Incomplete" right bundle-branch block. The configuration is exactly like full-blown right bundle-branch block except that the QRS is clearly narrower — 0.11 seconds.

Why is this important? If there's an infarct involving the septum, the disappearance of a septal Q wave, with progression from "incomplete" to "complete" left bundle-branch block, may be the only ECG evidence of infarction. That was exactly the case in Figs. 5-7 and 5-8.

Intermittent Bundle-Branch Block

Complete, permanent bundle-branch block means that some part of a bundle branch is totally dead in functional terms. Sometimes cells in a bundle branch are injured but not totally dead — they're still capable of functioning. Injured cells in a bundle branch will often take an abnormally long time to recover after each transmission. In other words, the refractory period of the bundle branch may be abnormally prolonged.

You may see a pattern of bundle-branch block only on alternate beats (Fig. 5-9). This can produce a confusing pattern, as in Fig. 5-10. The trick here is to measure from the *beginning* of each QRS to the *beginning* of the next. That way the varying width of the QRS complexes won't confuse you. The QRS complexes in fact come exactly on time: The P wave of the narrow beat is hidden each time in the wide T wave caused by the bundle-branch block in the beat ahead of it.

Intermittent bundle-branch block can appear in more complex forms. In Fig. 5-11 there are two wide beats followed by a narrow beat in a pre-

FIGURE 5-7
Tracing on the day of admission for a suspected myocardial infract. Incomplete left bundle-branch block pattern is obvious with septal Q in I and avl.

cise pattern. These are all sinus beats with a consistent P-R interval. This is 3:2 intermittent bundle-branch block. One normal conduction is followed by two beats with bundle-branch block. This can simply mean a very prolonged refractory period in the diseased bundle branch or it may reflect more complex patterns with progressive partial penetrations of a bundle branch.

Normalizing Fusion

Remember ventricular fusion (Chap. 2)? It's what happens when a ventricular ectopic beat starts across the ventricle and collides with an impulse coming down through the AV node, so that the ventricles are activated by two impulses. The resulting beat will be hybrid in shape, somewhere between the normal QRS and the wide QRS of the VPC. The

FIGURE 5-8

Same patient, next day. The QRS is much wider (0.14 seconds) and the septal Q has disappeared. This was strong confirmatory evidence of acute ischemic change involving the septum.

FIGURE 5-9

Lead V1. 2:1 right bundle-branch block. The refractory period of the right bundle branch is so prolonged that it can conduct only every other beat.

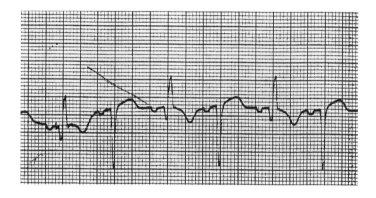

FIGURE 5-10

2:1 bundle-branch block. To recognize what's happening, it's important to measure from the beginning of each QRS complex — in fact they all measure out exactly despite the varying widths.

FIGURE 5-11

3:2 bundle-branch block. The refractory period is so prolonged that the malfunctioning bundle branch can conduct only on every third beat.

FIGURE 5-12

Mechanism of normalizing fusion. When bundle-branch block is present, a ventricular ectopic beat may sometimes activate the blocked ventricle at the same instant that the other ventricle is activated normally, thus producing a normal, narrow QRS by accident.

P-R interval will always be *shorter than normal* because the VPC begins to be inscribed while the normal impulse is still up in the AV node.

Fusion beats tell you that the wide complexes without P waves that you see somewhere else in the tracing have to be VPCs because the only way two impulses can collide, or fuse, in the ventricles is for one impulse to start in the ventricles in the first place. When you see fusion beats during a wide-beat tachycardia, the diagnosis is ventricular tachycardia, with 100% accuracy. That's why fusion beats are important.

Here's an unusual kind of fusion you can see when bundle-branch block is present. Suppose a ventricular ectopic impulse fires in the blocked ventricle. Suppose also that by pure coincidence the VPC activates the *blocked* ventricle at the same instant that the normal impulse coming down from the AV node activates the other ventricle. Both ventricles will be activated at the same fraction of a second and the QRS will be narrow. The bundle-branch block will disappear, for no apparent reason, for one beat (Fig. 5-12).

In other words, this is a kind of fusion that "normalizes" a bundle-branch block. The P-R interval of the "normalized" beat will be shorter

FIGURE 5-13
Lead I. Normalizing fusion. In the middle of each strip there's a narrow QRS preceded by a short P-R — a typical example of normalizing fusion.

FIGURE 5-14
Lead V1. Normalizing fusion in the setting of atrial fibrillation. Left bundle-branch block is present, and there's an ectopic focus firing in the left ventricle, producing the occasional wide beats. Beat four is narrow, obviously the result of normalizing fusion.

than normal, just like any fusion beat. When you see a normal QRS interrupting a bundle-branch block for no apparent reason, it means there's a ventricular ectopic focus firing, "normalizing" the bundle-branch block. These "normalized" beats may be your only clue to ventricular ectopic firing in the presence of bundle-branch block; that's why it's important to recognize them (Figs. 5-13 and 5-14).

Fascicular Blocks, or Hemiblocks; Bifascicular and Trifascicular Blocks

The left bundle branch isn't the simple structure physicians used to think it was. About twenty-five years ago investigators found that the left bundle branch has two distinct functional elements that conduct in different directions. If you dissect out the left bundle branch by special techniques, it looks like a fan with a long narrow handle: You can't make out any separate pathways or channels anatomically.

Functionally, the story is totally different. The left bundle branch behaves as if it had two different functional elements, conducting in roughly opposite directions. These functional elements are called *fasci-*

FIGURE 5-15

Schematic representation of the direction of conduction of the two fascicles of the left bundle branch.

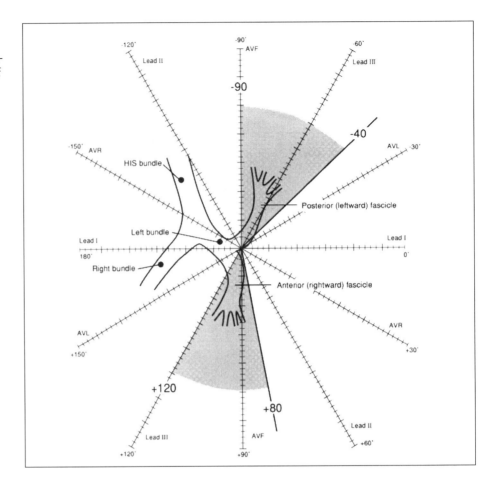

cles. The two fascicles are named according to the direction they conduct in, thus there is a posterior-superior, or leftward, fascicle and an anterior-inferior, or rightward, fascicle. The posterior-superior fascicle conducts upward and to the left at an angle of about −60° (range −40° to −90°). The anterior-inferior fascicle conducts downward and to the right at an angle of about +100° (range +80° to +120°) (Fig. 5-15).

When both fascicles are conducting normally, they balance each other out with a normal axis in the range of +30°. When one fascicle fails because the cells are diseased or dead, the axis will swing far to the left or right, with unopposed conduction down the functioning fascicle. Thus if the anterior fascicle fails there will be unopposed leftward conduction and the axis will lie between −40° and −90° (Fig. 5-16).

Logical question: Can anything else swing the axis this far left? Not much. Left ventricular hypertrophy or a high diaphragm in a short, stocky person can produce an axis as far left as −30°, but it won't go beyond that. A few rare degenerative diseases, like cardiac sarcoid, may deviate the axis far to the left, but even in these cases it's possible that de-

FIGURE 5-16
Left anterior hemiblock
with axis of –55°. There is
also intraventricular delay
with a QRS of 0.10 to 0.11
seconds.

generation of the anterior fascicle may be the cause. As a general working statement it's fair to say that an extreme left axis as defined above usually represents anterior fascicular block.

The common term for fascicular block is *hemiblock.* This isn't a very precise term since it implies that half of the bundle branch is blocked. In fact the anterior fascicle is much smaller and more vulnerable than the posterior fascicle — possibly a quarter of the size. However, the term *hemiblock* is in common use, so it's acceptable. The conclusion from all this is that left anterior hemiblock is a relatively precise, positive diagnosis, based on axis.

It was formerly argued that there must be a small, or "septal," Q in I and avl to establish the diagnosis of left anterior hemiblock, but this notion has been substantially discarded. It's the axis that establishes the diagnosis. Left posterior hemiblock is trickier. Posterior hemiblock will produce an extreme right axis, in the range of +80° to +120°, but so will many other conditions: right ventricular hypertrophy, pulmonary hypertension (acute or chronic), a tall slender habitus, or emphysema (Figs. 5-17 and 5-18).

Only when all other reasonable causes of an extreme right axis have been ruled out can you consider posterior hemiblock as a cause of right axis deviation. Posterior hemiblock is therefore a diagnosis of exclusion.

Remember, you have to correct for age and body habitus when considering axis. It's normal for children and young people to have a right

FIGURE 5-17
Physiologic right axis deviation of +100° in a tall, slender, young individual.

FIGURE 5-18
Pathologic right axis deviation of +112° appearing in a stocky, middle-aged individual early in the course of a myocardial infarction. Posterior hemiblock was the diagnosis of exclusion once a pulmonary embolus had been ruled out.

axis; on the other hand, if a slightly obese 65-year-old with otherwise normal heart and lungs turned up with a +90° axis, the only reasonable diagnosis would be posterior hemiblock. Posterior fascicular block is rare, presumably because the posterior fascicle is the larger of the two fascicles, with a more secure blood supply.

Special clinical significance: If a fascicular block of either variety appears abruptly in the course of an infarct, it may be a sign of acute ischemic change in the septum.

Fascicular blocks and AV conduction: In terms of AV conduction, fas-

FIGURE 5-19
Bifascicular block. The right bundle branch is blocked, as is the anterior fascicle of the left bundle. Conduction now depends exclusively on the posterior fascicle of the left bundle.

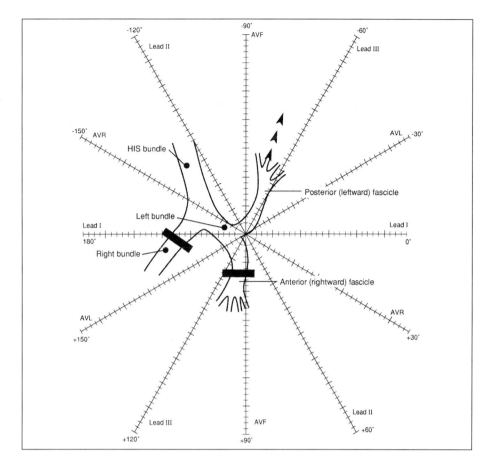

cicular blocks by themselves have no significance. In other words, the appearance of fascicular block does not present a significant risk of subsequent AV block. There's only one situation in which you'd be concerned about fascicular block and AV conduction, and that's when fascicular block is associated with right bundle-branch block. (Left fascicular block couldn't be associated with left bundle-branch block, obviously, because if the whole bundle branch is blocked, there is no possibility of conduction down one of the fascicles.) Figure 5-19 makes the problem clear.

If there is right bundle-branch block together with block of one fascicle of the left bundle, the ventricular component of AV conduction is reduced to one strand out of three — the one remaining conducting fascicle of the left bundle. At this point the diagnosis is *bifascicular block.* Interruption or delay in this last remaining strand will produce some type of AV block.

How can you tell if one fascicle of the left bundle is blocked in the presence of right bundle-branch block? You do it by determining axis,

FIGURE 5-20
Method of measuring axis in the presence of right bundle-branch block. Since you're trying to determine conduction in the left bundle, it's important to measure axis at the time the left bundle is being activated, in approximately the first 0.06 seconds of the QRS.

FIGURE 5-21
Right bundle-branch block with left anterior hemiblock. Axis of initial 0.06 seconds is −55°.

just the way you do with ordinary hemiblock. Remember that you diagnose left anterior hemiblock by detecting extreme left axis deviation (–45° to –90°). That's exactly how you go about it when right bundle-branch block is present, with one difference: You ignore the wide terminal wave that represents "backward" movement across the blocked ventricle.

You want to know what the axis is when the impulse is coming down the left bundle — that's being recorded during the initial part of the QRS. You simply measure the axis of the initial 0.06-second forces of the QRS. That's the axis that's recorded when the impulse is moving down the left bundle and that's how you tell if one of the fascicles of the left bundle is blocked. Figure 5-20 shows how to do this.

When bifascicular block was first described, there was a widespread belief that if a patient presented with syncope and bifascicular block, it would be reasonable to investigate the possibility of intermittent AV block as a cause of the syncope. Studies over the last twenty years, however, have shown that bifascicular block isn't really much of a risk in terms of AV block. Bifascicular block is in fact fairly common, and the risk of progressing to AV block is small. Look at Figs. 5-21 and 5-22 and practice this simple measurement.

FIGURE 5-22
Right bundle-branch block with left posterior hemiblock. Extreme right axis of initial forces is present (+118°), and all other causes of right axis have been ruled out.

I-II-III   aVR-aVL-aVF   V1-V2-V3   V4-V5-V6

FIGURE 5-23

Trifascicular block. Prolonged P-R in the presence of right bundle-branch block and left anterior hemiblock. This always raises the possibility that the P-R delay is in the one remaining conducting fascicle — that is, in the posterior fascicle of the left bundle. While this tracing was being recorded the P-R interval prolonged dramatically, and a temporary pacemaker was inserted as the patient went into a high degree of AV block.

Trifascicular block means that there's some kind of delay or failure in the one remaining fascicle. Thus if you saw bifascicular block with a prolonged P-R interval, it would be possible that the delay might be in the one functioning fascicle, and *trifascicular block* would be the appropriate term (Fig. 5-23).

Nonspecific Intraventricular Conduction Delay

Sometimes you'll see widened QRS complexes that don't fit the definite pattern of any kind of bundle-branch block or fascicular block. The QRS will be 0.10 to 0.11 seconds wide, with no particular recognizable pattern. All you can use is the obvious term *nonspecific intraventricular conduction delay,* which is precisely what it is. There must be some slowing in the more distal arborizations of the bundle-branch system, but that's about all you can say. People used to play with terms like "local focal intraventricular block," but they don't mean much in terms of real pathophysiology. Appearance and disappearance of this kind of delay, of course, may be a clue to acute changes, ischemic or toxic, in the myocardium.

FIGURE 5-24
Intraventricular conduction delay in the setting of an acute posterior-lateral myocardial infarct. This kind of delay is sometimes referred to as *peri-infarction block.*

The term *peri-infarction block* has been used to describe the kind of non-specific conduction delay shown in Fig. 5-24. Intraventricular conduction had been normal previously; with the onset of a posterior-lateral infarct, the widened QRS appeared. It's tempting to call this a left anterior hemiblock, but note that lead II consists of a simple Q wave, while there are many smaller Q waves in other leads. It's probably inaccurate to try to estimate axis in the presence of pathologic Q waves, so the simple term *nonspecific intraventricular conduction delay* is a better description. Some part of the fascicular tissues must obviously be involved to produce a pattern like this. Figures 5-24 and 5-25 are examples of this kind of nonspecific delay in intraventricular conduction.

FIGURE 5-25
Intraventricular conduction delay. The QRS complexes are wide, but they're narrower than in true bundle-branch block (0.10 to 0.11 seconds). There's some slurring of the QRS in several leads, a common finding in this setting.

6

More About Aberrancy

The competent electrocardiographer must be ready to recognize aberrant conduction in any of its forms. Combinations of wide beats, narrow beats, and beats with changing morphology may present life-and-death decisions. Learning the mechanism of the various types of aberrant conduction is an essential drill, reminiscent of the "gimme 50 pushups" we used to inflict on recruits in 1942.

In Chap. 5 you learned about simple, "fixed" or permanent aberrancy. This can present as bundle-branch block, fascicular or bi- or tri-fascicular block and nonspecific intraventricular conduction delay.

Aberrancy is often transient. When it is, it will be the result of one of four mechanisms:

1. Simple prolongation of refractory period with rate-dependent aberrancy.
2. Ashman aberrancy.
3. Bradycardia-dependent aberrancy.
4. Random intermittent or "non-rate dependent" aberrancy.

Simple Prolongation of the Refractory Period with Rate-Dependent Aberrancy

In Fig. 3-4 you saw a simple example of rate-dependent bundle-branch block. The same phenomenon can produce any of the other conduction defects listed above. Thus you may see rate-dependent fascicular blocks or rate-dependent intraventricular conduction delay (Fig. 6-1). The logic remains clear: There is normal conduction up to a certain rate and the aberrant conduction appears at any higher rate.

Simple prolongation of refractory period can produce regular ratios of conduction, like the 2:1 or 3:1 bundle-branch block illustrated in Figs. 5-7, 5-8, and 5-9. The concept remains the same: The refractory period is so prolonged that the structure can conduct only every other beat or every third beat.

FIGURE 6-1
Lead II. Rate-dependent intraventricular block — left anterior hemiblock. Throughout most of the tracing the QRS complexes are 0.11 seconds wide and show a left axis of approximately –45°. At the right-hand end of each strip, there is a pause after a premature atrial beat; after the pause a narrow QRS is apparent (0.08 seconds) with a normal axis. This is an obvious case of rate-dependent block in the fascicular system.

Ashman Aberrancy

There's another common form of aberrancy, called *Ashman aberrancy* after the man who described it.

To understand Ashman aberrancy you have to understand three simple facts:

1. The refractory period of the tissues of the heart depends on the *rate.* The slower the rate, the longer the refractory period after each beat. As the rate speeds, the refractory period shortens. (If you think about it, it has to, or the heart couldn't speed up very much.) See Fig. 6-2.
2. The refractory period of the heart is set *one beat at a time.* In other words, the refractory period after any beat depends on the distance between that beat and the beat ahead of it — the "rate" as far as any given beat is concerned is the distance from the beat ahead of it. Therefore, if the distance between beats varies, the way it does in atrial fibrillation and other arrhythmias, the refractory period will also change from beat to beat.
3. This changing refractory period sets up conditions for Ashman aberrancy. Look at the bottom strip of Fig. 6-2. Start with a long R-R interval. This means that there will be a long refractory period after the second beat of the pair. Now suppose the next beat comes early: There's a short R-R interval after a long one. The early beat will hit the refractory period set by the long R-R interval. Obviously, it will be blocked or aberrantly conducted. Thus when you see a short R-R interval following a long one, look for aberrant conduction (Fig. 6-3).

FIGURE 6-2
The mechanism of the Ashman phenomenon.

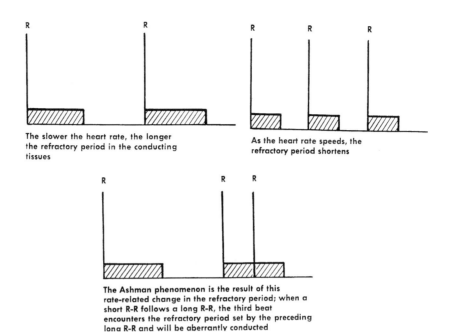

The slower the heart rate, the longer the refractory period in the conducting tissues

As the heart rate speeds, the refractory period shortens

The Ashman phenomenon is the result of this rate-related change in the refractory period; when a short R-R follows a long R-R, the third beat encounters the refractory period set by the preceding long R-R and will be aberrantly conducted

FIGURE 6-3
Ashman aberrancy in premature atrial beats. The premature beat provides the short R-R interval, which sets up the classic Ashman relationship.

When there's a run of rapid beats, as there is in a paroxysmal supraventricular tachycardia, the second beat in the run is the one that's likely to show Ashman aberrancy because of the long R-R/short R-R relationship. The short R-R then "pulls in" the refractory period, and beats from then on are normally conducted. This is the "second beat in the run" phenomenon, typical of Ashman aberrancy (Fig. 6-4).

One of the common settings for Ashman aberrancy, of course, is atrial fibrillation, or flutter with varying AV conduction, since there are changing R-R intervals with every beat. This helps with the problem of wide beats appearing during either arrhythmia. Are they aberrantly conducted beats from the atria or are they VPCs? If the wide beats appear when there's no Ashman ratio to explain them, they have to be VPCs! See Fig. 6-5.

FIGURE 6-4
Ashman aberrancy during paroxysms of atrial tachycardia. Each time there's a wide aberrant QRS it comes when a short R-R interval follows a much longer one. The two arrows point to the third and fourth beats in a run of atrial tachycardia. Note that while the second beat in the run shows Ashman aberrancy, the subsequent beats have normalized because the continuing short R-R intervals have "pulled in" the refractory period.

FIGURE 6-5
Diagnosing ventricular ectopic beats by excluding any basis for aberrancy. You can't make out any Ashman relationship with the wide beats — in fact they usually follow a long R-R interval instead of a short one. You can't invoke rate-dependent aberrancy either, because the wide beats come at a much slower rate than many of the narrow beats. The wide beats therefore must be ventricular.

Moral: When you see wide beats during atrial fibrillation or flutter with varying AV conduction, look at the R-R interval of the two beats ahead of them. If there's not a long R-R interval ahead of the wide beats, you can't call the wide beats aberrant. They have to be VPCs.

Delayed Ashman Reset
If a tachycardia is very fast compared to the basic rate, it may take several seconds for all parts of the conducting system to reset the refractory period — that is, to shorten it. For this reason you may see wide beats in a sustained run at the beginning of a tachycardia, then narrow beats ap-

FIGURE 6-6
Delayed Ashman reset. The strip starts with a sinus rhythm with a rate of about 90. A supraventricular tachycardia with a rate of 187 appears: The first seven beats are wide (arrows), after which the tachycardia continues with narrow complexes at exactly the same rate. This is the same Ashman phenomenon except that it's delayed. When the rate is rapid, it often takes several seconds for the refractory period to "reset" to normal in all parts of the conducting system. If you saw only the first seven beats, it would be easy to confuse this with ventricular tachycardia. The fact that the narrow complexes continue to appear at exactly the same rate as the wide ones tells you they must all be coming from the same place: they're supraventricular.

pear at exactly the same rate. The fact that all the beats appear at the same rate means they're all coming from the same place, of course. It's simply the Ashman phenomenon prolonged for a few seconds. Precisely why this occurs has never been explained. It may be because some parts of the ventricular conducting network aren't penetrated for the first few beats, and hence their refractory period isn't shortened (Figs. 6-6 and 6-7).

It's important to be aware of the possibility of delayed Ashman reset because it can produce wide-beat tachycardias that look exactly like ventricular tachycardia. Look for the normalized QRS complexes that appear at the same rate!

Special note: Rate-dependent aberrancy will produce a left-bundle branch configuration about 8 times out of 10. Ashman aberrancy will produce a right bundle-branch pattern about 8 times out of 10.

Phase 4 Aberrancy, or Bradycardia-Dependent Aberrancy

The idea of aberrancy that occurs because the impulse is coming too fast is simple. You can also see aberrancy when impulses come too slowly. Here's how it works:

Think of a conducting cell as an archer. Between beats, the bow is bent with the arrow drawn clear back. The cell is charged with *negative* energy, ready to release it. The energy is about –90 millivolts. It's potential energy, just like the bent bow. When the cell is activated, the energy is released, exactly like an arrow taking flight. The energy level in the cell goes down from –90 to about +10. After discharge, the cell is quiescent, passive — just like a bow after a shot. There's no potential energy. Then the cell recharges itself, like the archer drawing the bow for the next shot. It will recharge itself to about –90 millivolts.

FIGURE 6-7
Runs of supraventricular
tachycardia with delayed
Ashman reset, as in the
case above. In the top
strip, there'd be no way to
tell that the wide-beat
tachycardia wasn't ventricular. In the bottom three
strips you see typical delayed Ashman reset with
normalization of the QRS
after several seconds. Note
that the axis swings dra-
matically as the QRS com-
plexes narrow, suggesting
varying refractoriness in
the fascicular system.

Suppose our archer had to wait too long for the next shot. His arm gets tired, and he lets the bow go down to the half-drawn position. If he shoots from that position, it's going to be weak. The same thing can happen in conducting cells. Under certain conditions, *when there's a long time between beats,* the cells "leak" their charge, maybe to –50 millivolts. If they're stimulated at that low level of energy they will fire weakly or maybe not at all.

The phase of cell activation between beats is called "phase 4": That's when the cell should be at full charge, ready to fire. If the cells leak their charge during that period, it's called *phase-4 depolarization* or *bradycardia-dependent aberrancy.* Figures 6-8 and 6-9 are examples of this interesting and sometimes baffling phenomenon.

FIGURE 6-8
Bradycardia-dependent bundle-branch block. In most of the leads you see an obvious left bundle-branch block at a rate of 68. In leads V4, 5, and 6 there are normal narrow QRS complexes at a rate of 88. You can see the same thing in the rhythm strip at the bottom, with wide complexes at a slower rate and narrow complexes when the rate speeds.

FIGURE 6-9

Serial tracings. Marked sinus arrhythmia with one blocked premature atrial beat (at the right-hand end of the top strip). When the rate speeds to 88 the QRS is normal. Whenever it slows, a bundle-branch block is present. Typical bradycardia-dependent aberrancy is present.

Random, Intermittent, "Non-Rate-Dependent" Aberrancy

This is the rarest form of aberrant conduction. In Figs. 6-10 and 6-11 you see a bundle-branch pattern that appears and disappears at exactly the same rate as the normal beats. There's no Ashman phenomenon, no phase 4 mechanism, no rate change at all. The bundle-branch block simply appears and disappears in random fashion. This will always be the

FIGURE 6-10
Random, non-rate-dependent bundle-branch block. Lead V1, atrial tachycardia. Obvious right bundle-branch block pattern in the first portion of the tracing with normal intraventricular conduction in the second half. The rate is identical throughout and there is obviously no change in rhythm.

FIGURE 6-11
Random, non-rate-dependent aberrancy. Lead V1. Right bundle-branch block changing to normal QRS at the same rate (100). Note the interesting progression from complete to "incomplete" right bundle-branch block for one beat in the transition to normal intraventricular conduction.

result of some intermittent acute change in the conducting tissues as a result of drug effect, electrolyte intoxication, or ischemia. When this type of random conduction defect appears, one should always check for a possible cause, since it implies a changing, unstable condition in the conducting tissues.

Self-Assessment I

FIGURE I-1

1. The patient came to the emergency room with an obvious anterior MI. He received thrombolytic therapy and shortly thereafter this rhythm appeared.
   a. Diagnosis of wide-beat rhythm?
   b. Diagnosis of arrhythmia in the second strip?
   c. Is AV block present?
   d. Treatment?

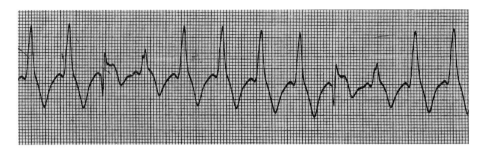

FIGURE I-2

2. Wide-beat tachycardia.
   a. Where does it originate? How do you know?

FIGURE I-3

3. Narrow-beat bradycardia.
   a. Where does it originate?
   b. Why?

FIGURE I-4

4. What are the diagnostic possibilities here?
   a. Can you distinguish between them?
   b. How will you treat this arrhythmia?

FIGURE I-5

5. Wide-beat tachycardia with two differing morphologies, lead V1.
   a. Diagnosis of arrhythmia?
   b. How proved?
   c. This all appeared in the setting of an acute MI in a patient with a previously normal ECG. Significance? Prognosis?

FIGURE I-6

6. This rhythm appeared in a critically ill postoperative patient. (CSP refers to "carotid sinus pressure.")
   a. What's happening and why?
   b. Possible effect on hemodynamics?

FIGURE I-7

7. Wide beats, narrow beats, and intermediate beats.
   a. Diagnosis? Proof?

FIGURE I-8

8. Wide beats and narrow beats.
   a. What are the wide beats?
   b. What's their pathophysiologic basis?

FIGURE I-9

9. Wide beats and narrow beats.
   a. What are they and why are they happening?

FIGURE I-10

10. Wide beats, narrow beats, and abrupt pauses.
    a. Why the variation in QRS width?
    b. Why the abrupt pauses?

FIGURE I-11

11. Sinus rhythm interrupted by a four-beat run of wide and narrow beats.
    a. What's the cause of the tachycardia?
    b. What's the pathophysiology of the changing QRS width?

FIGURE I-12

12. Somebody saw these wide beats in the emergency room and called for lidocaine.
    a. What's really going on?
    b. Pathophysiology of differing wide QRS morphology?

A

B

FIGURE I-13A and B   13. Both strips represent the same arrhythmia.
        a. Diagnosis?
        b. Cause?
        c. Treatment?

FIGURE I-14   14. Lead II. Interesting change in morphology of QRS throughout this tracing. It appeared early in the course of an MI. (Hint: remember this is lead II; think *axis!*)
        a. Cause?
        b. Significance?

FIGURE I-15   15. Arrhythmia? Cause of pause?

FIGURE I-16

16. Dramatic change in QRS morphology.
    a. Cause?
    b. Significance?

A

B

FIGURE I-17A and B

17. Two examples of supraventricular tachycardia: one in short paroxysms, one sustained.
    a. Cause in each?

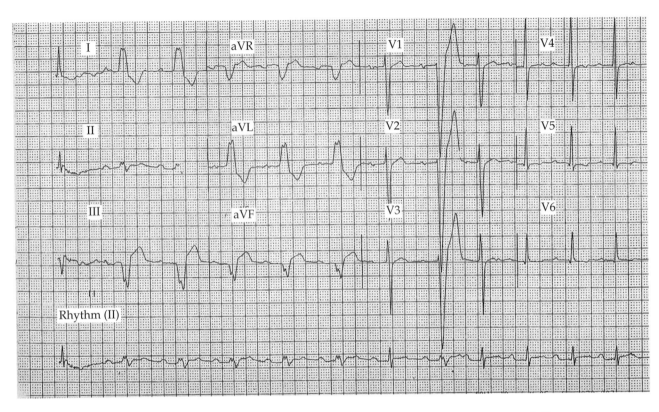

FIGURE I-18

18. Wide beats, narrow beats. What's the basis for the difference?

FIGURE I-19

19. Rhythm?
    a. Why is it present? What's lacking?

I-II-III   aVR-aVL-aVF   V1-V2-V3   V4-V5-V6

Rhythm [II] 5mm/mV (Auto)

FIGURE I-20

20. Easy. This tracing is recorded in an asymptomatic patient preoperatively.
   a. Diagnosis? Significance?
   b. Treatment if any?

FIGURE I-21

21. Both leads are V1. They're sequential.
   a. What's the wide-beat tachycardia in the top strip? Could it possibly be junctional with aberrancy?

FIGURE I-22

22. Note the abrupt slowing of rhythm.
    a. Cause?
    b. Treatment, if needed?

FIGURE I-23

23. Here's a rare and dangerous bird. What do you note about the wide-beat tachycardia?

FIGURE I-24

24. Comment on the wide beats. What's the mechanism that produces them?

FIGURE I-25

25. Comment on the wide beats. What's the mechanism that produces them?

FIGURE I-26

26. This rhythm appears in a 16-year-old who's been complaining of "fast palpitations" for years.
    a. Diagnosis?

Answers

1. The wide beats represent an accelerated idioventricular rhythm: Note fusion in the next-to-last beat in the bottom strip. The idioventricular rhythm "escapes" whenever the sinus rate falls below 60. In the second strip there is complete AV dissociation but there is no — repeat *no* — AV block. This is simple "interference-dissociation." No treatment needed.

2. Ventricular tachycardia. Note pairs of narrow beats. One is a complete capture beat and the next is a fusion beat. Infallible diagnosis!

3. Accelerated junctional rhythm. Note prominent retrograde P waves. This retrograde conduction will of course suppress the sinus node unless it accelerates to a rate faster than the rate of the junctional focus.

4. Two possibilities: ventricular tachycardia or junctional tachycardia with bundle-branch block. You can't possibly make the distinction. *Treat as ventricular:* You may help and you can't hurt.

5. The first 4 beats on the top strip are sinus beats with right bundle-branch block. This is followed by a wide-beat tachycardia with dissociated P waves; the same rhythm persists through the first 4 beats of the bottom strip. Dissociated P waves mean that the wide-beat tachycardia is almost certainly ventricular. Beat 5 in the bottom strip is a fusion beat: infallible diagnosis of ventricular tachycardia!

6. Accelerated idiojunctional rhythm in the first six beats. Carotid sinus stimulation suppresses the junctional focus and allows the sinus node to take over. In this critically ill patient resumption of sinus rhythm with "atrial kick" was lifesaving, so atropine was

administered followed by atrial pacing. Curious fact: Carotid sinus stimulation affects junctional foci more than the sinus node.

7. Runs of ventricular tachycardia. In the bottom strip you see four wide beats without P waves, followed by an obvious fusion beat. In the top strip *all the ventricular beats are fused:* The sinus node happens to be going about as fast as the ventricular rhythm so that there's fusion of every beat.

8. Premature atrial beats with Ashman aberrancy. Note the premature P waves tucked away in the preceding T waves.

9. Rate-dependent bundle-branch block with nonconducted premature atrial beats. Sometimes the pause after the PAC is long enough to allow normal intraventricular conduction to resume.

10. Frequent premature atrial beats with Ashman aberrancy. Look closely at the T wave ahead of the wide beats and you'll see that it's different from the T wave of the preceding beat. There has to be a P wave hidden in it. In the second strip the premature atrial impulses are frequently blocked; note the T wave ahead of each pause and you'll note the different shape due to the P wave hidden in it. In this critically ill patient the slowing was life-threatening: Blocked PACs can be a dangerous "brake" on the sinus node.

11. Supraventricular tachycardia with delayed Ashman reset. The wide beats and the narrow beats come at precisely the same rate, so they must be coming from the same place — they're all supraventricular.

12. Runs of paroxysmal atrial tachycardia with Ashman and rate-dependent aberrancy, producing, respectively, right and left bundle-branch patterns of aberrant conduction. Note again the phenomenon of delayed Ashman reset in the fourth, fifth, and sixth beats in the bottom strip.

13. Multifocal atrial tachycardia. Note dramatic changes in P wave morphology and rapid rate. This is always associated with chronic lung disease with hypoxemia. (In our institution, in addition to restoring oxygenation we've been using IV magnesium with about a 70% success rate.)

14. Rate-dependent left anterior hemiblock. Note that axis swings to about –60° with the slightly wider beats; when the rate slows, the QRS complexes are narrow with a normal axis. Appearing acutely in an MI, this of course suggests an acute process involving the septum.

15. Two premature atrial beats with a long P-R: The premature P wave is hidden in the preceding T — look at the small notch on the T.

16. Alternating right and left bundle-branch block. This means that there's dysfunction of both bundle branches, with real danger of total failure of AV conduction. Intervention urgent!

17. A. Obvious AV nodal reentrant tachycardia. Note that each short paroxysm begins with a PAC with prolonged P-R. Note also the retrograde P waves with varying relation to QRS — typical of a reciprocating process.

    B. Paroxysmal supraventricular tachycardia. This could be AVNRT or there could be a concealed bypass tract — you can't tell from this tracing alone.

18. The wide beats appear when the rate slows, the narrow beats when it speeds. Bradycardia-dependent aberrancy.

19. Junctional rhythm, rate about 38, with retrograde P waves. What's lacking? Sinus P waves, of course! There's no evidence of sinus node activity, hence the escape automatic rhythm functioning in its physiologic, lifesaving mode.

20. Right bundle-branch block with left anterior hemiblock. We used to worry about asystole during anesthesia or surgery but it turns out we didn't need to. No extraordinary measures are needed before or during surgery.

21. There's a wide-beat tachycardia with a right bundle-branch block configuration. This is followed by normal sinus rhythm with *left bundle-branch block.* The tachycardia must be ventricular; the alternative explanation of junctional tachycardia with right bundle-branch block is impossible. To have a pattern of right bundle-branch block you have to have conduction down the left bundle branch. Since the left bundle branch doesn't conduct at all, this is impossible.

22. Two VPCs with retrograde conduction to the atria. The retrograde conduction discharges the sinus node and produces the pause that permits the escape of the junctional focus. If this pattern is repetitive with a slow rate that compromises hemodynamics, it's necessary to eliminate the cause — the VPCs.

23. Rare and dangerous form of ventricular tachycardia. Note the alternating amplitude of the wide complexes. This is ventricular tachycardia with electrical alternans, a very dangerous, near-terminal digitalis-toxic rhythm.

24. VPCs. They're interpolated, meaning there's no postectopic pause. They're also *reentrant* — note the fixed coupling interval that continues for many repetitions.

25. VPCs, parasystolic. Note the wide variation in coupling to the preceding sinus beat. Note also that these beats appear at a fixed interectopic interval of about 480 milliseconds.

26. True ectopic atrial tachycardia. Note the well-defined P waves with different morphology from the sinus P. (This type of tachycardia is notoriously resistant to drug therapy; ablation as a means of treatment is very promising.)

7 | AV Block: Where Is It Localized and What Do You Do About It?

Sites of AV Block

Start with the picture in Fig. 7-1. In any consideration of AV block you begin with the fact that the AV conducting system consists of two distinct, well-defined elements:

1. The AV node–His bundle complex.
2. The proximal portion of the bundle-branch system.

The cells in the AV node are different in structure and function from the cells down in the bundle branches. They discharge and recover differently. When they fail, the pattern of abnormal conduction is different, and so is the prognosis.

Thus when AV block of any kind appears, it may be crucial to determine which element has failed. If you were a mad scientist and wanted to block conduction from atria to ventricles, the simplest way to do it would be to cut or poison the AV node. At this site AV conduction — and often life itself — depends on a single strand of tissue. Down in the bundle-branch system the task would be more complicated. If you cut

FIGURE 7-1
The possible sites of AV block. Failure of AV conduction may be localized in the AV node (n) or in the proximal parts of the bundle branches (b). Note that AV conduction in this area will not be interrupted unless *both* bundle branches fail.

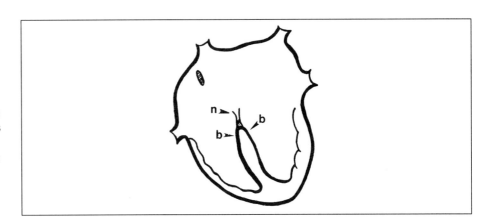

only one bundle branch you wouldn't interrupt conduction from atria to ventricles. You'd produce bundle-branch block, but as the reader already knows, AV conduction would continue down the other bundle with no delay. To interrupt conduction from atria to ventricles you'd have to cut *both* bundle branches. Thus only when both bundle branches are malfunctioning will you see failure of AV conduction in the bundle-branch system.

This may all seem obvious, but it's critical to some of the diagnoses you're going to learn to make in this chapter.

How to Localize Block and How to Classify It

The first step in logic is to determine the degree of AV block. AV block is rationally and usefully divided into first-, second-, and third-degree block. (A little while back, when invasive electrophysiologic studies were in first bloom, some cardiologists suggested that these three classic categories were obsolete: In fact they have emerged as more useful than ever.)

In *first-degree block* every atrial impulse reaches the ventricles but takes longer than normal getting there. The P-R interval is *fixed.* Anything over 0.20 seconds should be considered prolonged in the adult heart.

In *second-degree block* some atrial impulses reach the ventricles while others are blocked. Second-degree block may come in one of three forms:

1. Type I or Wenckebach block. This is the most common form of second-degree block, and for practical purposes, it's always located in the AV node.
2. 2:1 or other "fixed ratio" block, such as 3:1 or 4:1. This may be localized in the AV node or in the bundle-branch system.
3. Type II or Mobitz-II block. This is always — repeat *always* — located in the bundle-branch system.

Third-degree block means complete heart block with no transmission from atria to ventricles. It may be localized in the AV node or in the bundle-branch system.

Now try combining these items into specific diagnoses. Figures 7-2, 7-3, and 7-4 are all obvious examples of first-degree AV block. Where's the block? Look at the QRS complexes. They're *narrow.* A narrow QRS means that both bundle branches are functioning normally. The AV delay cannot possibly be located in the bundle-branch system: It must be up in the AV node.

FIGURE 7-2

First-degree AV nodal block, P-R 0.41 seconds.

FIGURE 7-3

First-degree AV nodal block, P-R 0.24 seconds.

FIGURE 7-4

First-degree AV nodal block. In the upper strip the P is completely hidden in the T. In the lower strip the P can be seen as a notch coming off the peak of the T. P-R interval approximately 0.32 seconds.

Rule: When you see narrow QRS complexes, any failure of conduction must be located in the AV node. It cannot possibly be located in the bundle-branch system. (To imagine first-degree AV block with a narrow QRS localized in the bundle-branch system you would have to imagine absolutely identical delay, to the thousandth of a second, in the two separate bundle branches — an obviously absurd idea.)

Now consider Fig. 7-5. Bundle-branch block is present, and there's a prolonged P-R interval. In this case you can't tell where that delay is taking place. There's a single strand connecting atria and ventricles; it con-

FIGURE 7-5
First-degree AV block with
left bundle-branch block.
AV conduction now de-
pends on a single func-
tional strand consisting of
the AV node and the right
bundle branch (arrows).
The delay in AV conduc-
tion could be taking place
anywhere along that
strand; you can't localize it
from this tracing.

sists of the AV node and the one functioning bundle branch. The delay
may be taking place anywhere along that strand — that is, in the AV
node or in the bundle branch. You can't tell the difference from this tracing alone.

The difference here is not significant. First-degree AV block, no matter
where it's localized or how prolonged the P-R, is never a threat to life,
and no intervention is required.

Common error: Sometimes I hear residents commenting that "the P-R
is too long to be conducted" when the P-R interval is in the range of 0.40
to 0.50 seconds. That of course, is nonsense: Prolonged P-R intervals of
0.60 seconds and even higher have been recorded. If you see a fixed P-R
in a series of beats you can be certain the atrial impulse is reaching the
ventricles. It would be statistically impossible for two independent pacemakers to coincide within a hundredth of a second and produce a fixed,
sustained, P-R relation.

An occasional problem with first-degree block is illustrated in Fig. 7-6.
The P-R interval may be so prolonged that the P is hidden in the preceding T. You can see a "bump" on the T in the top strip that strongly suggests a P wave: To be certain, simply slow the rate by having the patient
rest or by applying carotid sinus stimulation. When the rate slows, the P
will move out of the T (see Fig. 7-6, bottom strip).

FIGURE 7-6
First-degree AV nodal block unmasked by carotid sinus stimulation. In the top strip you can't tell whether or not there's a P wave hidden in each T. By stimulating the carotid sinus, slowing the sinus and producing temporary AV nodal block, the clinician can unmask the hidden sinus P waves, making it clear that this is indeed a sinus rhythm with first-degree AV nodal block. P-R approximately 0.40 seconds.

The Three Types of Second-Degree Block

Type I, or Wenckebach, Block

There are five defining characteristics in Type I block. They're all based on the character of AV nodal cells. These cells are activated by a slow inward current, and when they're diseased or intoxicated, they show *progressive fatigue* ending in failure of conduction, with subsequent recovery.

The five specific characteristics of Type I block are as follows:

1. Progressive prolongation of P-R intervals. To document this you have to see two or more consecutive P-R intervals, of course. This seems obvious, but it's surprising how often physicians lose sight of it.

2. Failure of conduction with a blocked P after maximum P-R prolongation.

3. Recovery with shortening of P-R interval after the blocked P wave.

4. A pause after the blocked P that is *less than the sum of the two beats before the blocked P.* This has to be the case since the P-R always shortens after the blocked P; naturally, this shortened P-R "pulls in" the QRS so that it comes relatively early: The pause has to be less than the sum of the two preceding beats.

5. R-P/P-R reciprocity. The sinus P waves keep coming at a fixed rate while the P-R prolongs. Obviously each QRS is going to be "pushed out" closer to the next P (simple arithmetic!). Thus there's a reciprocal relation between R-P and P-R. To put it another way, the closer each P wave comes to the preceding QRS, the more fatigued the AV nodal cells will be (because they've had less time to recover) and the longer the next P-R will be. Again, this seems obvious, but you'll use it to solve some complex problems.

Figure 7-7 is an example of "typical" Wenckebach block. The maximum prolongation of P-R takes place in the second beat of the cycle with

FIGURE 7-7
Typical Wenckebach block with progressive prolongation of P-R before the blocked P. (The blocked P is hidden in the T of the beat before the pause.) The pauses are always less than the sum of the two preceding beats because the P-R after the pause always shortens.

FIGURE 7-8
"Atypical" Wenckebach block with maximum prolongation of P-R in the last conducted beats and many junctional escape beats (J). The junctional focus here, of course, is performing its normal "escape pacemaker" function.

much smaller increments in subsequent beats. Where's the blocked P? Put your calipers on the P waves and you'll see that it's buried in the T wave of the last beat of the cycle. This is a common and sometimes confusing phenomenon. Look for all the other criteria of Type I block.

If you measure the R-R interval carefully, you'll notice a curious phenomenon: Although the P-R interval grows longer, the R-R interval shortens a little. This is because the amount of prolongation of the P-R is less with each beat even though the total P-R is longer. The P-R intervals in Fig. 7-7 start at 0.28 then jump to 0.32 in the second beat, 0.36 in the third, and 0.39 in the fourth. The R-R interval will actually shorten *since the degree of increase of the P-R is less* with each beat. Try it with a ruler and you'll see how it works. This is the "Wenckebach paradox" of shortening R-R when the P-R increases by diminishing increments. It's present in what is loosely termed "typical" Wenckebach block — maybe in 70% to 80% of all cases. If you remember this characteristic R-R shortening, it will help you recognize Type I block in some unusual settings.

Figure 7-8 illustrates "atypical" Wenckebach block. There's minimal prolongation of P-R until the last beat of the cycle, when it prolongs abruptly. This tracing also illustrates a common complication of Type I block. After the blocked P waves, there are junctional escape beats that at one point form a sustained idiojunctional rhythm.

Figure 7-9 shows 3:2 Wenckebach block, meaning that two beats are conducted while a third is blocked. Note that this forms a paired, or "bigeminal," rhythm.

2:1 or "Fixed Ratio" Block

The tracing in Fig. 7-10 takes the reader into the next pattern of conduction: "fixed ratio" block. Every other P wave is conducted with a fixed P-R interval, while the alternate P wave is blocked. You call this exactly what it is: 2:1 block. 2:1 block with a narrow QRS is of course located in the AV node.

Figure 7-11 illustrates both 2:1 and Wenckebach block in the AV

FIGURE 7-9
3:2 Wenckebach block. The blocked P is seen as a notch in the T before the pause. Note that the 3:2 ratio of conduction produces a paired, or "bigeminal," pulse.

FIGURE 7-10
2:1 AV nodal block. Note the fixed relation of P to QRS throughout.

FIGURE 7-11
2:1 AV nodal block changing to a 3:2 Wenckebach cycle in the right-hand side of the strip. This is a common combination in AV nodal block.

node — a frequent combination. It's common to see 2:1 AV nodal block vary with Wenckebach periods since both types of block are really manifestations of the same AV nodal dysfunction.

2:1 AV BLOCK WITH BUNDLE-BRANCH BLOCK. This form of block (Fig. 7-12) is much more disturbing. Since one bundle branch is permanently blocked, the block of the alternate P waves might be taking place in the other bundle branch. In other words, this might represent *intermittent bilateral bundle-branch block.* It might also represent coincidental AV nodal block. You can't tell which from this tracing alone.

Figure 7-13 shows another example of "fixed ratio" block with bundle-branch block. In this case the ratio is 4:1. Note that the P-R interval of the conducted beats remains the same, just as in 2:1 block. Again, the failure of conduction might reside in the AV node or in the one functioning bundle branch. There's no way to make the distinction from this tracing.

Rule: When you see 2:1 or other "fixed ratio" block with a narrow QRS, it means that the block is in the AV node. It's relatively benign and may be caused by drugs such as digitalis, beta blockers, or calcium blockers or by transient ischemia.

FIGURE 7-12
AV block with bundle-branch block. If the block is in the AV node, it's relatively benign. On the other hand, if it's in the bundle branch, there is *intermittent bilateral bundle-branch block,* a very dangerous situation. The need for pacing is urgent. You can't tell the difference from this ECG.

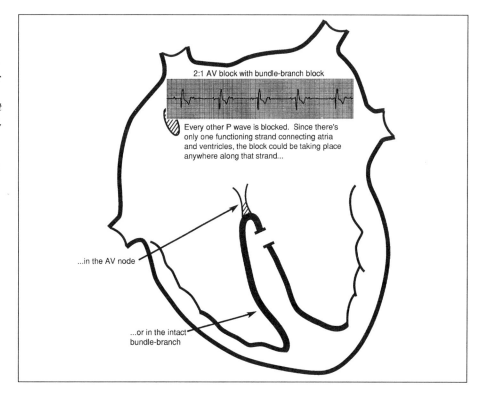

2:1 AV block with bundle-branch block

Every other P wave is blocked. Since there's only one functioning strand connecting atria and ventricles, the block could be taking place anywhere along that strand...

...in the AV node

...or in the intact bundle-branch

FIGURE 7-13

4:1 AV block with bundle-branch block. Note the absolutely fixed relation of P to QRS throughout. Since you don't see two consecutive P-R intervals anywhere, you can't localize the block precisely. But a rate this slow will always produce CNS or cardiovascular symptoms, and intervention will be needed.

FIGURE 7-14

Mobitz-II block with intermittent periods of 2:1 AV block. If all you saw were the two periods of 2:1 block in the left half of the strip you couldn't localize the block, but the periods of 3:2 block on the right side tell you this block is localized in the one functioning bundle branch. Pacemaker!

When you see "fixed ratio" block with a wide QRS, it raises the possibility that you're looking at intermittent bilateral bundle-branch block. This is potentially very dangerous. It will never be the result of such drugs as digitalis, although it can be the result of transient ischemia.

How to make the distinction between block in the AV node and block in the other bundle branch? This introduces the third category of second-degree block: Mobitz Type II.

Type II or Mobitz-II Block

In Fig. 7-14 you see some periods of 2:1 block with a wide QRS (part of the QRS is almost hidden in the baseline but it's really 0.12 seconds wide). You also see periods like the three beats in the middle where there are two consecutive conducted beats followed by a blocked P — in other words, 3:2 block. Now you can diagnose the location of the block with absolute accuracy. During the period of 3:2 block you see the following:

1. Two consecutive conducted beats with the same P-R (no Wenckebach type of prolongation).
2. A blocked sinus impulse.
3. A P-R interval in the first beat after the block with the same P-R interval as the beats before.
4. A pause around the blocked P equal to exactly twice the sinus rate.

You have made an absolute diagnosis of Mobitz-II block. That's all you have to see. What you're looking at is in fact intermittent bilateral bundle-branch block. You will see Type II block only in the presence of preexisting bundle-branch block. It never takes place in the AV node.

During the periods of 2:1 conduction, of course you couldn't be sure of the location of the block. Until you see two *consecutive* conducted beats you can't be sure the 2:1 block won't slide into Type I periods as in Fig. 7-11. Those two consecutive beats with a fixed P-R make the diagnosis for you; the other findings confirm it.

Type II block carries a very grave prognosis. The risk of catastrophic asystole is about 36% per year. Mobitz-II block is an absolute indication for permanent pacing. You don't wait for symptoms: The first symptom is likely to be the last symptom that a patient ever experiences — especially if the asystole appears while the patient is driving a car!

Mobitz-II block is misunderstood more than any other abnormality of rhythm or conduction.

Figure 7-15 gives a diagrammatic representation of Mobitz-II block. Type II block is a result of the electrophysiologic characteristics of

FIGURE 7-15
Schematic representation of Mobitz-II block. Study this carefully. This is the most misunderstood phenomenon in electrocardiography and one of the most important. In Mobitz-II, the failure of conduction will always be abrupt. There is *no* warning prolongation of the P-R interval before the blocked P wave, and there is *no* shortening of the P-R interval in the first beat after the blocked P wave. Everything stays the same except that one or more P waves are suddenly not conducted. This kind of all-or-none conduction is seen only in the bundle branches, never in the AV node.

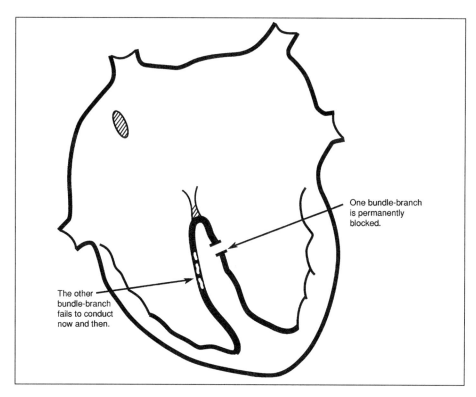

One bundle-branch is permanently blocked.

The other bundle-branch fails to conduct now and then.

FIGURE 7-16
3:2 Mobitz-II block. As always, bundle-branch block is present, the consecutive P-R intervals are constant, and the pauses are an exact double of the basic rate.

FIGURE 7-17
2:1 AV nodal block with period of 4:3 Wenckebach block. Contrast this with the Type II block in Fig. 7-16.

FIGURE 7-18
Mobitz-II block produced by atrial pacing. The pacer spike precedes the P wave. All the features of Type II block are present: the fixed P-R throughout and the pauses that equal a double sinus interval. (The QRS is really 0.12 seconds wide — this tracing has been reduced, and part of the QRS is hidden in the baseline.)

bundle-branch cells. They depend on the fast inward sodium current for activation, and when they fail they fail abruptly. It's all-or-nothing conduction, just like rate-dependent bundle-branch block. This is in sharp contrast to AV nodal cells, which always show progressive fatigue and recovery.

Figure 7-16 is a typical example of Type II block with a 3:2 ratio of conduction. Note the elements of Type II block.

Figures 7-17 through 7-22 are examples of Type I and Type II block with wide and narrow QRS complexes. Try diagnosing each of them and compare your results with the legends.

FIGURE 7-19
Mobitz-II block in the setting of right bundle-branch block with left anterior hemiblock. The block is taking place in the posterior fascicle of the left bundle.

FIGURE 7-20
Wenckebach block with bundle-branch block. It's perfectly possible to have AV nodal block in the presence of bundle-branch block and that's what you see here. All the characteristics of Wenckebach block are present, and it would be exceedingly rare to see this happening down in the one functioning bundle branch. This was in fact digitalis-toxic AV nodal block.

FIGURE 7-21
3 : 2 Wenckebach block
with sinus bradycardia.
Regardless of the site of
block, the effective rate is
so slow that the patient
will certainly experience
symptoms and some inter-
vention will be needed.
This case was not drug-
induced or transient, and
permanent pacing was re-
quired.

FIGURE 7-22
Wenckebach block. Con-
trast this and Fig. 7-21
with Figs. 7-16, 7-17, 7-18,
and 7-19 and the difference
between Type I and Type
II blocks becomes obvious.

Complete Heart Block

The diagnosis of complete heart block is based on three elements:

1. Complete AV dissociation with no capture beats — in other words, complete absence of AV conduction.
2. A ventricular rate of 45 or less.
3. A sufficient number of atrial impulses to probe all aspects of diastole.

Special note: The ECG diagnosis of AV dissociation is based on two simple yes-or-no questions:

1. Is there a changing relation of P to QRS? If yes:
2. Is the ventricular rhythm regular despite this changing P-R relation-ship? If yes:

AV dissociation is present. Obviously the P waves and the QRS complexes have nothing to do with each other. Their relation is accidental, like a di-vorced couple passing in the street.

Figure 7-23 is a schematic illustration of complete AV block. In this pa-tient, the block is localized in the AV node — note the narrow QRS. (I've had many staff ask me if AV nodal block can be complete, and of course

FIGURE 7-23
Complete AV nodal block. Ventricular rate 34. Complete AV dissociation: ample numbers of sinus P waves but none come through to "capture" a beat. Conclusion: No conduction is possible.

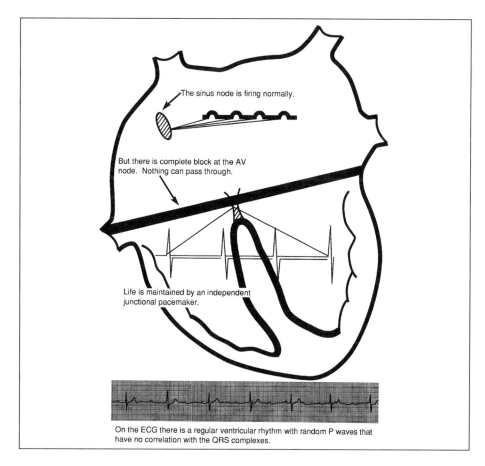

The sinus node is firing normally.

But there is complete block at the AV node. Nothing can pass through.

Life is maintained by an independent junctional pacemaker.

On the ECG there is a regular ventricular rhythm with random P waves that have no correlation with the QRS complexes.

the answer is "yes," just as illustrated here. AV nodal block can be complete and life-threatening.)

Note the term *AV dissociation.* Most physicians aren't very clear about what it means and what forms it comes in. It's time to stop and differentiate the two types of AV dissociation. One is common and harmless, the other is rare and dangerous. (After almost fifty years of teaching this subject I know that AV dissociation ranks right up there with Mobitz-II block in the great misapprehension derby. This is not the fault of the medical profession at large; the language used to describe this simple phenomenon has been so complex and the definitions so vague that I'm reminded of the instructions with the E-Z assembly toys we all struggled with at 1 A.M. on Christmas morning.) Therefore we now define AV dissociation and describe the two causes and types.

Definition: Complete AV dissociation means that the atrial and ventricular rhythms are separate and independent. The atria are driven by one pacemaker — usually the sinus node — while the ventricles are driven by an ectopic focus in the node or in the ventricles. The two rhythms have nothing to do with each other. They're divorced.

Complete AV dissociation is not the same as complete AV block. In fact, about 99% of the time it has nothing to do with AV block. A good example of the common type of AV dissociation is the kind you see in some cases of ventricular tachycardia (Chap. 3). The ventricular tachycardia keeps bombarding the AV tissues so rapidly that they're refractory to any sinus impulse.

In this case the AV dissociation is caused by the "interference" of the ectopic rhythm. The proper name for this kind of dissociation is *interference-dissociation*. You can see interference-dissociation any time an ectopic rhythm in the node or the ventricles fires rapidly enough to make the tissues refractory to the sinus impulses. In simple terms, the ectopic focus gets in the way of the sinus impulse. There's nothing wrong with the AV conducting tissues; there's no block (Fig. 7-24).

Figures 7-25 through 7-31 are all examples of interference-dissociation. Take some time with them and become thoroughly familiar with this harmless and much-misunderstood arrhythmia.

FIGURE 7-24
Interference-dissociation. The atrial and ventricular rhythms are dissociated because of the "interference" of an ectopic focus in the node or the ventricles that fires just fast enough to make the AV tissues refractory whenever a sinus impulse arrives.

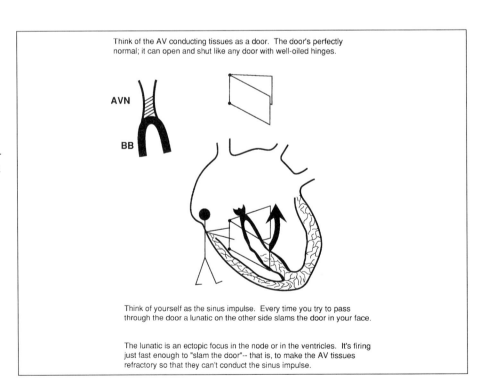

Think of the AV conducting tissues as a door. The door's perfectly normal; it can open and shut like any door with well-oiled hinges.

AVN

BB

Think of yourself as the sinus impulse. Every time you try to pass through the door a lunatic on the other side slams the door in your face.

The lunatic is an ectopic focus in the node or in the ventricles. It's firing just fast enough to "slam the door"-- that is, to make the AV tissues refractory so that they can't conduct the sinus impulse.

FIGURE 7-25

Interference-dissociation. A normal sinus rhythm is interrupted by a junctional rhythm (sixth beat) that fires a little faster than the sinus node and keeps the AV node refractory. The P waves gradually disappear into the QRS.

FIGURE 7-26

Intermittent interference-dissociation. The first three beats are idioventricular beats. In the fourth beat the sinus node "gets ahead" of the ectopic focus and captures the rhythm for three beats (c). The sinus rhythm and the accelerated idioventricular rhythm compete throughout the strip with periods of dissociation and periods of capture by the sinus node. During the idioventricular rhythm the sinus P waves are buried in the QRS, but you can march them right out with the capture beats.

In Fig. 7-25 there is a series of normal sinus beats interrupted by a junctional rhythm that fires a little more rapidly than the sinus node, forming the dissociated pattern of the last five beats.

In Fig. 7-26 the predominant rhythm is an accelerated idioventricular rhythm dissociated from the sinus rhythm. The beats marked "c" represent capture by the sinus node when it fortuitously arrives at the AV node between ectopic beats. (Note the fusion beat marked "f.")

AV Block: Where Is It Localized and What Do You Do About It? **101**

FIGURE 7-27
Interference-dissociation caused by an accelerated junctional rhythm (round black dots in the diagram). The junctional rhythm is faster than the sinus rhythm (75 versus 63), so the junctional beats "interfere" with the sinus beats most of the time. There are occasional sinus capture beats (C) when the sinus impulse arrives at just the right time between ectopic beats.

In Fig. 7-27 the dissociation is caused by a junctional rhythm firing a little faster than the sinus node, while in Figs. 7-28 and 7-29 the dissociation is produced by an accelerated idioventricular rhythm discharging at almost the same rate as the sinus node. Figures 7-30 and 7-31 are again examples of interference-dissociation caused by a junctional rhythm discharging faster than the sinus node.

Study these well. They were all mistakenly diagnosed as AV block, and in several cases pacemakers were proposed!

FIGURE 7-28
Interference-dissociation caused by an accelerated idioventricular rhythm with a right bundle configuration (left side of strip). Beginning with the first beat marked "C," the sinus node begins to capture the ventricles with progressive fusion with the ectopic focus. The last two beats on the right show that there's really a left bundle-branch block.

FIGURE 7-29
Interference-dissociation caused by the discharge of an idioventricular pacemaker. The sinus impulses, labeled "P," march through the idioventricular rhythm until they cycle out ahead of the ectopic focus and capture the rhythm.

FIGURE 7-30
Interference-dissociation caused by a combination of sinus bradycardia (rate 53) and an accelerated junctional rhythm (rate 62). Most of the beats are junctional with an occasional sinus capture (C).

FIGURE 7-31
Interference-dissociation caused by an accelerated junctional rhythm discharging at almost the same rate as the sinus node. In the middle part of the strip, the sinus and junctional rhythms are almost identical ("isorhythmic").

FIGURE 7-32
Complete AV nodal block. There is complete AV dissociation with no capture beats, and the ventricular rhythm is set by a pacemaker in the junction with a rate of 45. There are P waves appearing all through diastole, far from the junctional beats, yet none are conducted — thus the effect of "interference" is ruled out.

Now you're ready for the definitive diagnosis of complete heart block. In Fig. 7-32 you see complete AV dissociation. Next you see a ventricular rhythm of about 48. Finally you note that there are P waves occurring all through diastole. There's plenty of time between those ectopic QRS complexes for an atrial impulse to come through and capture the rhythm if the AV system were capable of conducting. The slow rate of the rhythm driving the ventricles rules out any question of interference. The diagnosis is complete AV block. The narrow QRS tells you the block is in the AV node.

Figures 7-33 and 7-34 are both examples of complete AV nodal block. Examine each for the criteria listed above.

FIGURE 7-33
Complete AV nodal block with a ventricular rate of 28. This is an example of life-threatening complete block in the AV node.

FIGURE 7-34
Complete AV nodal block, ventricular rate 39. Note that all the criteria for complete AV block are present.

FIGURE 7-35
Complete AV block in the bundle-branch system with an idioventricular rate of 32. This patient was a young woman who suffered from congenital primary fibrous degeneration of the myocardium. It is interesting to note that she attended high school and carried on a relatively normal life with this slow rate in the era before pacemakers. She finally died of congestive heart failure, not of asystole.

FIGURE 7-36
Complete AV block, ventricular rate 39. The wide ventricular complexes could represent an idioventricular rhythm or a junctional rhythm with bundle-branch block. You couldn't tell the difference from this tracing. Since the block was shown to be permanent, not drug-induced, the distinction became academic. Anyone with this degree of permanent block and this ventricular rate will need pacing, regardless of the site of the block.

In Figs. 7-35 and 7-36 you see complete heart block with wide ventricular complexes. There are two possibilities. First, the complete block may be the result of failure of both bundle branches — in other words, bilateral bundle-branch block. When the bundle-branch system fails, life can be maintained only by an idioventricular focus. Naturally the ventricular complexes are wide, like these. This might also be the result of complete AV nodal block with bundle-branch block, which would account for the wide complexes. The only way you could make the distinction would be to see a previous ECG with normal intraventricular conduction.

What's the difference whether the complete AV block is localized in the AV node or in the bundle-branch system? For one thing, block in the AV node is much more likely to be the result of drugs like digitalis, calcium blockers, or beta blockers. Digitalis and the calcium-blocking drugs have no effect on the bundle-branch system and the effect of beta blockers, if any, is negligible.

Block in the AV node is also much more likely to be the result of transient ischemic insult, such as the AV nodal block that accompanies inferior myocardial infarction. This specific kind of AV block is always ultimately benign. It always disappears, and permanent pacing is never needed.

On the other hand, complete block in the bundle-branch system carries a much graver prognosis. It can be a result of high potassium levels or, rarely, of tricyclic drugs, but in the vast majority of cases it represents intrinsic irreversible disease, and in such cases, pacing is always indicated.

If transient toxic or ischemic effects have been ruled out and complete AV block is permanent, the distinction becomes academic since permanent complete block with ventricular rates this slow will always require pacing in any case.

Before leaving this subject be sure you understand the following:

1. The five characteristics of Type I block.
2. The four characteristics of Type II block.
3. What "fixed ratio" block is.
4. The essential difference between AV nodal tissue and bundle-branch tissue when conduction is impaired.
5. How to diagnose AV dissociation.
6. The two causes of AV dissociation.
7. The three criteria for the diagnosis of complete heart block.
8. Special note: Don't forget that a shortening R-R interval is typical of the common form of Type I block. This phenomenon will help you recognize Type I block when there are no P waves — for instance, with Type I block around an automatic ectopic focus or with Type I block in the lower node in the presence of a junctional rhythm.

8

Diagnosis of Complex Forms of AV Block: Some Tricks, Some Booby Traps

"High Degree" of AV Block

The term *high-degree* is a good one for the kind of block illustrated in Fig. 8-1. There are many blocked P waves with only occasional conducted beats. There's no fixed pattern of AV conduction in the top strip: The paired beats may represent random paired firing from a junctional focus. In the bottom strip there's a consistent 4:1 ratio with a P-R of 0.52 seconds in the conducted beats. In other words, the term *high-degree block* is reserved for cases in which there are many blocked atrial impulses with occasional conducted beats, without any recognizable pattern of block.

"Pseudoblock"

The most common type of "pseudoblock" is illustrated in Fig. 8-2. Here there's a sinus rhythm with bundle-branch block. In the middle of both strips there's an abrupt pause. Look carefully at the T waves of the beats before each pause: They're obviously different from all the other T waves. There's a small "spiky" deformity just at the end of these T waves that you don't see in most of the other beats. At the left-hand end of the bottom strip you see a premature beat that's clearly

FIGURE 8-1
High degree of AV nodal block. Many blocked P waves in the top strip without any regular pattern of conduction. 4:1 block in the bottom strip.

FIGURE 8-2
Frequent nonconducted premature atrial beats. Occasional conducted premature atrial beats. Note the "glitch" in the T waves after the second beat in each strip. These are obvious nonconducted P waves.

supraventricular. In the T wave of the beat before this premature beat you see the same deformity.

These are obviously premature atrial beats superimposed on the T waves. One is conducted and the others aren't. Nonconducted or "blocked" premature atrial beats are the most common cause of pause in a sinus rhythm. (We put quotation marks around the term *blocked* because the word *block* really implies subnormal conduction. There's nothing wrong with the conducting apparatus here: the problem is that the premature P comes too early for anything to be conducted.)

Rule: When you see an inexplicable abrupt pause, always look at the T wave ahead of the pause to see if there's a premature, nonconducted P wave hidden in it. Remember Isaiah's rhetorical question: "Doth the leopard change its spots?" Of course it doesn't, and in the same way the T wave doesn't change its shape from beat to beat. When you see a change in the shape of a T wave it practically always means there's a P hidden in it.

The nonconducted premature atrial impulse is wasted motion; it discharges the sinus node but it doesn't itself reach the ventricles — hence the pause. The nonconducted PAC acts as a "brake" on the sinus node.

The tracing in Fig. 8-3 was actually misclassified as Mobitz-II block and the patient was scheduled for a permanent pacemaker. The combination of right bundle-branch block and left anterior hemiblock certainly provides the right setting for Mobitz-II block, and there is in fact

FIGURE 8-3

A nonconducted premature atrial beat producing an abrupt pause in a patient with bifascicular block (right bundle-branch block with left anterior hemiblock).

an abrupt pause in the sinus rhythm. At this point you apply the rule and remember Isaiah. The T wave of the beat ahead of the pause is clearly different in shape from all the other T waves. There has to be a P wave hidden in it — no other explanation. You're simply looking at a nonconducted premature atrial impulse. There's no significant failure of AV conduction. If you look at the second beat ahead of the pause, you'll notice that it comes early, with a prolonged P-R . Thus there are two premature atrial beats, one conducted and one blocked. The patient doesn't need anything except reassurance.

Figure 8-4 is a tracing recorded early in the course of a myocardial infarct. Many wide QRS complexes appeared, some in runs, and there was the usual rush to lidocaine with the notion that the wide beats were ventricular.

To analyze this arrhythmia look first at the fifth beat in the bottom strip. This shows what a normal sinus beat should look like. Now look at the first beats in each strip; each is followed by a premature atrial impulse. In the top strip the premature atrial beat produces a sharp negative deflection in the T wave and it's not conducted. In the bottom strip the premature atrial beat produces a large upright P and it is conducted with Ashman aberrancy. Look throughout both strips and you'll see

FIGURE 8-4

Multiple premature atrial beats — some blocked, some conducted with Ashman aberrancy. Note how easy it would be to confuse this with ventricular ectopic discharge. See text for precise analysis.

FIGURE 8-5

Frequent premature atrial beats — some conducted with Ashman aberrancy, some blocked. The blocked PACs in this case produced a slowing of effective rate that jeopardized the patient's life.

these premature atrial beats in the T waves; sometimes they're not conducted, but when they are you see typical Ashman aberrancy — long R-R preceding short R-R. The final diagnosis is therefore "frequent premature atrial beats, some conducted aberrantly, some blocked." No ventricular ectopy, no need for lidocaine.

In Fig. 8-5 the same phenomenon became life-threatening. Early in the course of a severe myocardial infarction some wide beats and some long pauses appeared. When the rate was 80, the blood pressure was barely maintained; during the pauses when the rate fell to the low 40s, the pressure plummeted and the patient was quickly in distress. Every treatment but the right one was proposed: pacing (useless), atropine (useless), isoproterenol (lethal).

Again, look at the T waves ahead of the pauses. They're obviously different from the sinus T waves: There's a sharp, "spiky" element, very different from the flat, almost isoelectric sinus T. Blocked PACs are deforming the T waves; the nonconducted premature atrial impulses are producing the pauses. If you look at the T in front of the occasional wide beats you also see a premature P deforming the T. These are conducted

FIGURE 8-6
High degree of AV block
with long pauses around
the frequent VPCs. The
"interference" of the VPCs
is actually exacerbating the
effect of the block, with
many long pauses.

premature atrial beats, and the wide beats are simply another example of Ashman aberrancy.

If blocked PACs slow the heart rate critically, as they do here, what do you do? You treat the PACs, of course. You use drugs that suppress ectopic activity in the atria. Digitalis and quinidine are probably best; digitalis would be preferred in an acute situation because it can be given by vein. Blocked premature atrial beats cause the only bradyarrhythmia that is treated with suppressive drugs. The suppressive drug (digitalis) worked swiftly and completely in this case: The PACs disappeared and the sinus rate of 80 was maintained.

(Note: When you make this diagnosis and prescribe this treatment you'll be met by incredulous stares. This particular case was reviewed at the Arizona Heart Annual Scientific Session on two successive years by Drs. Bernard Lown and H. J. C. Marriott. One recommended digitalis, the other quinidine! Stick to your guns and ignore the possibly lethal recommendations of the uninformed.)

Figure 8-6 presents a case of very significant block made functionally much worse by the presence of VPCs. There's really a sinus tachycardia with a rate of 125. Many of the P waves are hidden in the QRS, as you'll see if you use the calipers. The AV block is complex.

Basically, these are Wenckebach periods, with 2:1 block at some points and many junctional ectopic beats. The wide QRS is cause for concern about possible Mobitz-II block, but there are no true Type II patterns anywhere.

There are many long pauses when the effective rate drops to about 36. Note that these pauses always occur around a VPC. There's always a P wave just ahead of the VPC and one shortly after it. Neither atrial impulse can be conducted because of the interference of the VPC. The P wave just ahead of the VPC obviously doesn't get a chance to reach the ventricles, and the one after the VPC finds the AV conducting tissues refractory from the effect of the VPC on the bundle-branch tissues and the AV node.

Retrograde conduction of VPCs up the AV node is very common and often produces prolonged refractoriness with subsequent block of the sinus impulse. Always take this effect into consideration when you're analyzing AV block. Eradicating VPCs can often reduce the degree of block or eliminate it entirely.

Pseudo-Mobitz-II Block: Concealed His Bundle Beats

If you see what looks like Mobitz-II block with narrow QRS complexes, take another look. It probably isn't Mobitz-II block. For practical purposes, Mobitz-II block is always found in the setting of preexisting bundle-branch block.

In Fig. 8-7 the tracing certainly looks like Type II block. There are fixed P-R intervals with occasional blocked sinus P waves. There's no change in the P-R after the blocked P. Why isn't this Mobitz-II block?

If you look elsewhere in the tracing you see that many junctional premature beats are "sandwiched" between sinus beats, or to use a more scientific term, they are "interpolated." (While these beats may arise in the His bundle, I use the term "junctional" because it's more familiar and the effect is exactly the same.) There's no pause after them. That means that they were not conducted retrogradely across the atria; they didn't reset the sinus node. In other words, there is retrograde block to the junctional beats. Every now and then there is also antegrade block. The ectopic focus in the junction or the His bundle fires and makes the tissue refractory, but you never see it. The only way you can tell it happened is that the next sinus impulse is mysteriously blocked.

Figure 8-8 is another example of the same phenomenon. There are obvious junctional beats (J). There are occasional blocked P waves, with the same P-R after the block as before. Note that the junctional beats labeled "J" are not conducted retrogradely — you know that because the next sinus P comes on time. Exactly when the next junctional beat should come, you see a blocked sinus P wave. This isn't real block: It's a form of interference caused by the discharge of the ectopic focus in the junction or the His bundle. This discharge is totally blocked, as illustrated in Fig. 8-9.

FIGURE 8-7

Concealed His bundle beats producing a "pseudo-Mobitz-II phenomenon." This is a very old tracing that may look a bit fuzzy, but it's a classic example. In the top two strips you see many junctional beats (J) interpolated between two sinus beats. These beats don't interrupt the sinus rhythm, which means they're not conducted back across the atria. There's retrograde block. In the third strip, right where the junctional beat should appear, you see a blocked P. It looks like Mobitz-II block because there's no Wenckebach prolongation of P-R ahead of the blocked P and no shortening of P-R after it. What's really happened is that the junctional focus wasn't conducted backward *or* forward. All it did was make the node refractory so that the P wave wasn't conducted. Harmless!

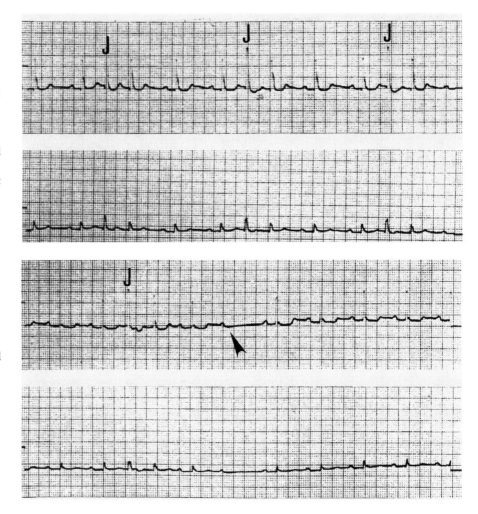

FIGURE 8-8

Frequent concealed His bundle or junctional beats mimicking Type II block. There are frequent junctional beats often occurring in pairs. The sinus P waves march right through them so you can tell that the junctional beats aren't conducted back across the atria. Exactly where the third junctional beat should occur, there's a blocked P.

FIGURE 8-9
Diagram of the effect of completely concealed firing in the His bundle or in the region of the junction. The ectopic focus fires (double arrows); even though it isn't conducted anywhere it leaves the tissue refractory. The P wave that comes just after this concealed firing is therefore not conducted. This can mimic Mobitz-II block, but in fact there isn't any block anywhere — there's only harmless interference. Junctional or His-bundle beats, concealed or not, don't mean anything and don't require treatment.

Moral: When you see what looks like Mobitz-II block with a narrow QRS, look around for interpolated junctional beats. This isn't Mobitz-II block: It's as harmless as any random junctional (or His bundle) beats.

The Langendorf-Pick Principle for the Diagnosis of Atypical Mobitz-II Block

Back to Wenckebach block for a moment. In Fig. 8-10 you see a 3:2 Wenckebach block. Start with the first QRS of the pair in the middle of the strip. Notice the distance to the next P, or the R-P interval. It's about 0.44 seconds. Look at the distance from the second QRS to the following P. It's much shorter, of course — about 0.22 seconds. In other words, there's a reciprocal relation between the P-R and the R-P in Wenckebach block. "Of course!" you exclaim. "Since the P-R gets longer it has to push the QRS out closer to each following P — after all, the P waves keep arriving right on time."

FIGURE 8-10
Typical Wenckebach block with 3 : 2 ratio. The distance from the first QRS of each pair to the following P wave (R-P interval) is much longer than the distance from the second QRS to the third P wave of the cycle. In other words, there is a reciprocal relation between P-R and R-P. This is characteristic of AV nodal block.

Think of the R-P as the rest period and the P-R as the working period. The longer a diseased AV node has to rest (R-P), the faster it conducts on the next transmission (P-R). When the rest period is shorter, the conduction will be slower. Down in the bundle-branch system, on the other hand, conduction is all-or-nothing. Consider rate-dependent bundle-branch block: the bundle branch is blocked or it isn't — nothing intermediate.

Now look at Fig. 8-11. In the top strip there's first-degree AV block with bundle-branch block. The P-R is 0.40 seconds. In strips 2 and 3, the block is 3:1, and in the bottom strip it's 4:1. This patient was taking digitalis — is this digitalis-toxic AV nodal block or is the block localized in the one functioning bundle branch?

You don't see two consecutive conducted beats anywhere, so your usual criteria for Type I and Type II block can't be used. What you do see, however, is a very wide change in the R-P interval. In the top strip the R-P interval is 0.52 seconds. In the strips with 3:1 block it's 1.64 seconds, and when the ratio goes to 4:1 it's 2.6 seconds. "R-P" here means the interval from the R to the next conducted P. Ignore the blocked P waves. Despite this dramatic change in the R-P, the P-R remains absolutely fixed. The block has to be in the other bundle branch. It's a variant of Mobitz-II block.

FIGURE 8-11
The Langendorf-Pick phenomenon. Rapid increase in degree of AV block in a patient with preexisting bundle-branch block. Note that no matter how long the R-P becomes, the P-R remains exactly the same. This is a variant presentation of Mobitz-II block.

With a degree of block this severe up in the AV node you would inevitably see striking changes in the P-R interval to correspond with the changing R-P. The P-R with 2:1 block would be a lot longer than the P-R with 3:1 block, and so on. This is an absolute distinction. You can count on it.

Figure 8-12 shows another example of the same phenomenon. This is lead V1; there's right bundle-branch block and there are many blocked P waves. In the top strip there is one junctional escape beat and then the rhythm settles down to 2:1 block. In the middle strip the ratio changes to 3:1 block, and in the bottom strip the 3:1 block is interrupted by one episode of 2:1 block. When the ratio changes from 2:1 to 3:1 there's obviously a very large change in R-P — from 1.6 seconds to 2.48 seconds to be exact — but the P-R remains absolutely fixed. This is a variant of Mobitz-II block, and the patient needs a pacemaker without further ado.

Figure 8-13 shows the opposite picture. In the top strip there's 3:1 block. In the middle strip there's complete block, and in the bottom strip the ratio shifts to 2:1 block with wide, aberrant ventricular complexes. The P-R with 3:1 block is 0.22 seconds, and the P-R in the bottom strip with 2:1 block is 0.39 seconds. See how dramatically the P-R changes in response to R-P change when the block is in the AV node? Even though there are wide QRS complexes, you can diagnose AV nodal block with complete confidence. All the patient needed was less digitalis!

Figure 8-14 shows R-P/P-R reciprocity in a little more complex setting

FIGURE 8-12
Lead V1: right bundle-branch block. The ratio of conduction changes from 2:1 to 3:1 throughout the tracing with corresponding drastic changes in R-P. Despite these changes the P-R remains absolutely fixed. Mobitz-II conduction! Pacemaker!

FIGURE 8-13
AV nodal block with changing P-R in response to changing R-P. Top strip, 3:1 block, P-R 0.21 seconds. Bottom strip, right-hand side, 2:1 block (with aberrant IV conduction); P-R 0.40 seconds. This is a variant of Type I AV nodal block. The diagnosis is precise.

FIGURE 8-14
R-P/P-R relation of AV nodal block manifested in the changing P-R of the capture beats (1, 2, 3, and 4). The P-R changes in precise reciprocal fashion with the R-P, thereby localizing the block in the AV node.

FIGURE 8-15
Solution to a perplexing clinical problem, namely 2:1 block with bundle-branch block. Where's the block? Answer: Run a lot of ECG paper looking for a change in the ratio of block!

(continuous strips). Basically, there's a dissociated junctional rhythm (J) with many blocked P waves. There are occasional capture beats (labeled 1, 2, 3, and 4). Look at the P-R intervals of the capture beats; they vary widely (beat 1, 0.28 seconds; beat 2, 0.32 seconds; beat 3, 0.36 seconds; beat 4, 0.40 seconds). Now look at the R-P intervals; they vary in an exact reciprocal pattern. The shorter the R-P, the longer the P-R of the capture beat, and vice versa. This is AV nodal behavior; all those P waves are being blocked in the AV node. (The narrow QRS is another giveaway in this case, but even if the QRS complexes were wide, what you see here would give you an absolute diagnosis of AV nodal block.)

"Well fine," says the harassed cardiologist, "but what if you have just plain 2:1 block with bundle-branch block? How can you tell what's going on?" Figure 8-15 gives one answer. Use plenty of ECG paper and wait for the ratio to change. Sometimes it changes spontaneously; more often it changes when the sinus rate slows. Record an ECG during sleep, when the sinus rate normally slows. Slow the sinus rate with carotid sinus pressure. Simply have the patient lie quietly so that the heart rate slows.

This patient came into the ICU with 2:1 block and bundle-branch block. The next day this tracing was recorded as the patient lay quietly in the ECG department. The 2:1 block changes to first-degree in the top strip and back to 2:1 in the bottom strip. In the bottom strip you see a classic Mobitz-II cycle as the ratio changes from first-degree to 2:1 — fixed P-R intervals, blocked P, resumption of conduction with unchanged P-R.

Before leaving this topic, look at Fig. 8-16. Which of these strips record Mobitz-II block? They were all diagnosed as possible Mobitz-II block. Stop here and analyze them yourself. In all five strips bundle-branch block is present.

FIGURE 8-16
Self-quiz (see text).

Strip A. Nonconducted premature atrial beat.

Strip B. Sinoatrial block with abrupt dropping of one sinus P wave.

Strip C. Typical Mobitz-II block.

Strip D. 2:1 block with bundle-branch block. Site of block cannot be determined; it could be in the AV node or in the other bundle branch.

Strip E. Mobitz-II block. The negative P waves are easily visible.

Intra-Hisian Block

This is a rare bird. When it became possible to record His bundle potentials it was discovered that in some cases there is a "split" His potential. That is, there are two separate potentials recorded during passage through the His bundle — one proximal and one distal. Block can take place within the His bundle itself, between the proximal and distal potentials. This block can produce an atypical Wenckebach cycle or, as reported in one case, a true Mobitz-II phenomenon.

Mobitz-II block within the His bundle is excessively rare: In over fifty years of studying electrocardiograms I've never seen a case. Intra-Hisian Wenckebach is probably more common. It's characterized by tiny incre-

FIGURE 8-17
Probable intra-Hisian block. Block within the His bundle itself may take the form of Wenckebach block with tiny increments of P-R , as here.

FIGURE 8-18
Probable intra-Hisian Wenckebach block with tiny increments in P-R before the blocked P.

ments in P-R interval, as shown in Figs. 8-17 and 8-18. Note how small the increases in P-R are in these tracings compared with AV nodal Wenckebach. Sometimes the increases are so small you can hardly measure them, but they do progress to block of one impulse and subsequent recovery. Nobody has any idea of the significance or prognosis of this kind of block. Presumably pacing would be indicated only if the ventricular rate became so slow as to compromise CNS or cardiovascular function in some way.

P Wave Shortage

Beware the great P wave shortage (Fig. 8-19). Remember that one of the criteria for complete heart block is "enough atrial complexes to probe all aspects of diastole." In this strip you start with complete AV dissociation in the first four beats. The ventricular rate is about 52. The last beat is a capture beat with a P-R of 0.23 seconds. Why the dissociation? *Measure the P-P interval and you find a sinus rate of 45.* That's the problem. The

FIGURE 8-19
Pseudoblock because of a
slow sinus rate. There's an
idioventricular rhythm
with complete AV dissoci-
ation for the first beats.
The reason for the idioventricular rhythm and the
dissociation is simply the
slow sinus rate.

sinus rate is so slow it lets an idioventricular rhythm escape with a rate
a little faster than the sinus node. This sets up the pattern of dissociation
that looks so alarming. There just aren't enough sinus impulses to test
the system. When one does arrive at a reasonable time after the "idio"
rhythm, it's conducted with nothing worse than first-degree AV block.
The patient had sinus bradycardia caused by clonidine. There was nothing significant wrong with the AV conducting system at all.

9

Atrial Fibrillation

Atrial fibrillation is the most common of the major disorders of rhythm. Most of you already know what's happening in the atria during fibrillation — that the atria are traversed by myriad very fine, rapid, irregular impulses that bombard the AV node like sparks flying off a pinwheel (about 450 impulses per minute in an average case). The ECG diagnosis of uncomplicated atrial fibrillation is remarkably simple:

1. There are no recognizable P waves.
2. There are usually fine, fast fibrillary waves with no consistent morphology.
3. The ventricular rhythm is irregular.

Note this last point: When the ventricles are responding to fibrillating atria, the ventricular rhythm will always be irregular — no exceptions.

(At this point it's important to dispose of a semantic myth. Students are taught that an "irregular irregularity" is diagnostic of atrial fibrillation. By this time the reader can probably think of three or four other arrhythmias that produce an "irregular irregularity," such as a pronounced sinus arrhythmia with a few premature beats, showers of ectopic beats from different foci, changing interplay of junctional and sinus rhythms, changing ratios of Type I block, and so on. Before the end of the book you'll be able to think of ten or more.)

There are several sources of confusion in the diagnosis of atrial fibrillation.

The Character of the Fibrillary Waves

Typical fibrillary waves produce fine, fast deflections in the base line that vary in shape and timing from second to second (Fig. 9-1). Sometimes they're obvious, but sometimes they're so small they're not visible.

FIGURE 9-1

Typical atrial fibrillation with characteristic "f" waves that appear and disappear. Note also the "pseudo–P wave" before the second beat: it's really just an isolated "f" wave.

FIGURE 9-2

Coarse atrial fibrillation, or flutter-fibrillation. The large, almost regular atrial complexes on the left side of the strip indicate a transient period of true flutter with an atrial rate of 300. They quickly dwindle into small fibrillary waves.

FIGURE 9-3

Coarse atrial fibrillation. The complete variability in shape and timing of the atrial complexes rules out flutter.

Figure 9-2 shows just how much these "f" waves can change. On the left-hand side they're perfectly regular, like flutter waves for a little while, and then they dwindle away and disappear. These fibrillary waves must not be confused with flutter, which is a sustained, mathematically regular atrial mechanism. If there's the slightest variation in shape or spacing of the "f" waves, the diagnosis is fibrillation, even though the "f" waves may be large and nearly regular.

Figure 9-3 is an excellent example of "coarse" atrial fibrillation, or "flutter-fibrillation." Note the large "f" waves at various parts of the tracing: They're almost regular for short periods. One more time: Do not confuse this with atrial flutter. The proper name is as above: "coarse atrial fibrillation" or "flutter-fibrillation." Prognosis and treatment are exactly the same as in any atrial fibrillation.

FIGURE 9-4
Flutter-fibrillation. Note that the atrial complexes are visible only in V1. They're too fast for flutter waves, which never exceed a rate of 300 in the adult. If you look closely you can also see minute changes in morphology — another feature that rules out flutter.

Figure 9-4 is a 12-lead tracing. Note that you can't even see fibrillary waves in any lead except V1, but here they're so coarse that they were mistakenly diagnosed as flutter. In fact, they're much too fast for flutter (about 450), and the morphology changes if you look at them minutely. Again the diagnosis is coarse atrial flutter or flutter-fibrillation, the latter an older but very descriptive term.

Figure 9-5 is another example of coarse fibrillation. (This particular phenomenon is described here at length because it's often confused with real flutter.)

What it you can't see any fibrillary waves, as in Fig. 9-6? You can still make a diagnosis with about 99% accuracy. No P waves plus an irregular ventricular rhythm equals a presumptive diagnosis of atrial fibrillation.

FIGURE 9-5
Flutter-fibrillation in a child. Note the coarse, almost regular atrial complexes that appear briefly on the left side of the tracing. This often confuses observers, but the proper diagnosis is coarse fibrillation or flutter-fibrillation.

FIGURE 9-6
Atrial fibrillation with one PVC. The fibrillary waves are so small they're invisible, but the absence of P waves and the totally irregular spacing of QRS gives the diagnosis.

Ectopic Beats

When the whole rhythm is irregular, it's often impossible to detect premature beating at the bedside. Obviously you can't have atrial premature beats if the atria are fibrillating. It is possible to have junctional premature beats interrupting atrial fibrillation, but it's difficult to recognize them even on an ECG, because the narrow junctional beats usually look exactly like the beats conducted from the fibrillating atria. There are two ways to recognize junctional ectopic beats during fibrillation; they're illustrated in Fig. 9-7.

First, the junctional beats may be aberrantly conducted, like the ones here (typical Ashman aberrancy). Second, and even more importantly,

FIGURE 9-7
Atrial fibrillation with two aberrantly conducted junctional beats. The two junctional beats are close to the preceding conducted beats. Inspection of the R-R intervals in the rest of the strip tells you that the AV node couldn't conduct that fast. The beats have to be reentrant junctional ectopic beats.

note that the two aberrant beats come much closer to the beats ahead of them than any two consecutive beats coming down from the fibrillating atria. In other words, it's obvious from looking at the rest of the tracing that the AV node couldn't conduct this fast. These early beats have to be the result of a reentrant ectopic focus.

The important ectopic beats are ventricular, of course. During an acute myocardial infarct they may be harbingers of fatal arrhythmias. They may also be an important early sign of digitalis toxicity (Chap. 16).

In Fig. 9-8 you see typical wide ventricular ectopic beats interrupting atrial fibrillation. How can you tell they're not aberrantly conducted impulses from the fibrillating atria? Apply the same criteria you did with the junctional beats. In the first place, the distance from the wide beats to the preceding conducted beat is shorter than any R-R anywhere else in the tracing. It's obvious the AV node couldn't conduct that fast, so these beats can't be the result of aberrant conduction from the atria. Furthermore, remember the rule about reentrant ectopic beats: They come at a relatively constant distance from the conducted beats that precede them (within a few hundredths of a second). This *constant coupling* to the preceding beats also rules out random conduction from the fibrillating atria.

Figure 9-9 is an example of a VPC interrupting atrial fibrillation. This wide beat might also be junctional with aberrancy. How do you make

FIGURE 9-8
Atrial fibrillation with ventricular ectopic beats. The short, consistent coupling interval of the wide beats to the preceding narrow beats rules out any possibility that the wide beats are the result of random aberrant conduction from the fibrillating atria.

FIGURE 9-9
Atrial fibrillation with one VPC. There's no possible basis for aberrant conduction, so the wide beat has to be ventricular.

the distinction? Simple: Look to see if there's any basis for aberrancy. In Fig. 9-9 the wide beat comes after a relatively long pause, so you rule out rate-related aberrancy. There is also no Ashman relationship, so there's simply no reason for aberrant conduction. The beat has to be ventricular.

Rule: You know the three causes of aberrant conduction. Don't diagnose aberrancy unless you see one of them.

These wide beats are VPCs. In the setting of an acute MI, reach for the lidocaine!

The Ventricular Rhythm Turns Regular

Of course this might mean that a normal sinus rhythm is now present. On the other hand, consider Fig. 9-10. The regular rhythm might come from an idioventricular rhythm like this one, firing just fast enough to "take over" from the fibrillary impulses for a time. The idioventricular rhythm is discharging at a rate of 90, and of course it's regular. While the idioventricular rhythm is present there is complete AV dissociation. None of the fibrillary impulses reach the ventricles. There's no block — remember, this is interference-dissociation caused by the discharge of an ectopic focus.

Rule: When the ventricular rhythm becomes regular during atrial fibrillation, it may be the result of complete AV dissociation with a junctional or ventricular rhythm driving the ventricles.

FIGURE 9-10
Atrial fibrillation with intermittent accelerated idioventricular rhythm. Note the fusion beat (F).

FIGURE 9-11
Atrial fibrillation interrupted by an accelerated idioventricular rhythm.

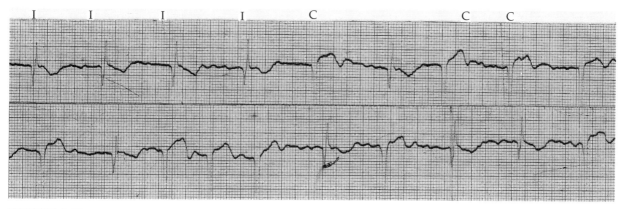

FIGURE 9-12
Atrial fibrillation interrupted frequently by short runs of an accelerated idiojunctional rhythm. The idiojunctional beats (I) form a complex pattern with the conducted beats from the fibrillating atria (C). The slow rate of the junctional rhythm (58) means that there must be some degree of AV nodal block.

Figure 9-11 shows another example of an accelerated idioventricular rhythm interrupting atrial fibrillation.

The interplay between the idiorhythms and the fibrillary impulses can produce some complex patterns, as in Fig. 9-12. The beats labeled "I" arise in the junction while the beats labeled "C" are conducted from the fibrillating atria. Moral: When you're examining a patient with known atrial fibrillation, listen carefully for any periods of regular beating. If there's the slightest question, record an ECG. Accelerated idiorhythms in the normal range are harmless; on the other hand, if they are slow, it's time to start thinking about heart block.

Look again at Fig. 9-12, for example. The rate of the idiorhythm is slow — about 58. There's plenty of time between ectopic beats for impulses from the fibrillating atria to come through the AV node if it were functioning normally, but obviously, it isn't: The idiorhythm controls the ventricles for long periods at a slow rate. There must therefore be a considerable degree of AV block. It's not complete because there are periods when the fibrillary impulses do reach the ventricles. This is therefore a type of second-degree AV block in the presence of atrial fibrillation. Some impulses reach the ventricles while others don't, even though they have plenty of time to do so. Since there are no P waves to measure from, this is as precise as you can be.

AV block in the presence of atrial fibrillation is very important because almost all patients with atrial fibrillation are taking some kind of medication that depresses AV nodal conduction. You must be alert to the possibility of significant heart block and detect it before it becomes life-threatening. Since there are no P waves you have to use simple logic, as above.

Criteria for AV Block in the Presence of Atrial Fibrillation

1. A slow but irregular heart rate (Fig. 9-13). Remember that the fibrillating atria are bombarding the AV node about 425–450 times a minute. If all the impulses reached the ventricles, of course, the patient would die quickly. Two things keep this from happening: the refractory period of the AV nodal tissue and the phenomenon of concealed conduction.

The effect of the refractory period on speed of conduction is obvious. The cells can't conduct until they recover from the previous transmission. "Concealed conduction" in this setting simply means partial penetration of the AV node by many impulses, with resulting fatigue of the nodal cells and a slower rate of conduction. A healthy AV node should conduct fibrillating impulses at a very rapid rate — up to 170–180. In older patients it's common to see slower conduction with normal ventricular rates.

FIGURE 9-13
Atrial fibrillation with slow ventricular rate varying from 43 to 68. The slow rate indicates a substantial degree of AV block; the irregular response indicates that it is not complete.

In Fig. 9-13, however, some of the R-R intervals are equivalent to a rate of 38, and the average rate is about 60. There must be a significant degree of AV block, although it's not complete.

2. Periods of AV dissociation with a slow "idio" rhythm — in the range of 55–65. As in Fig. 9-12, this means a high degree of block, less than complete.

3. Complete AV dissociation with a rate of 45 or less (Fig. 9-14). The rate is perfectly regular and there are no episodes of conduction from the fibrillating atria. The diagnosis is complete heart block. You use the same criteria you use for any complete heart block: complete AV dissociation with no capture beats, a slow ventricular rate, and enough atrial impulses to test the system all through diastole. (In atrial fibrillation there's a surplus of atrial impulses to do the testing!)

Atrial Fibrillation and Paroxysmal Tachycardia

When the rate becomes rapid and perfectly regular, in the range 140–240, paroxysmal tachycardia is interrupting the atrial fibrillation. The tachycardia may be junctional or ventricular.

Figure 9-15 is an example of junctional tachycardia; right bundle-branch block was present chronically. After periods of typical random conduction from the fibrillating atria, a regular rhythm appears for several seconds at a time. The rate is 150.

Rule: A rapid junctional rhythm in the high-normal to tachycardia range is the most common sustained digitalis-toxic tachyarrhythmia. When you see this type of arrhythmia in a digitalized patient, always assume digitalis toxicity (Chap. 16).

If a wide-complex tachycardia appears, it may be ventricular or junctional with aberrancy. Sometimes it's possible to make the distinction by using the same criteria you learned in Chap. 3:

1. Look for fusion beats. When the atria are fibrillating, there are so many impulses coming through the AV node that there are many

FIGURE 9-15
Atrial fibrillation interrupted by runs of paroxysmal junctional tachycardia (right bundle-branch block).

FIGURE 9-16
Atrial fibrillation interrupted by paroxysms of ventricular tachycardia. Note the striking progressive fusion beats and the end and the beginning of each episode of ventricular tachycardia.

chances for fusion. In Fig. 9-16 you can see the beginning and end of two paroxysms of ventricular tachycardia. The narrow beats in the middle of the strip represent the normal pattern of conduction. There is striking progressive fusion with the ventricular beats at the beginning and end of each run of tachycardia (f).

Figure 9-17 is another example. In Fig. 9-17A you see a simple wide-beat tachycardia. From this strip alone you can't make the distinction between junctional and ventricular origin. In Fig. 9-17B there are many obvious fusion beats as the rhythm changes to atrial fibrillation.

2. Look for a rate basis for aberrancy. Do the wide beats appear at a rapid rate and disappear when the rate slows? Fig. 9-17B gives an answer here as well. The narrow conducted beats appear at a rate *more rapid* than the wide L beats. Forget aberrancy!

FIGURE 9-17

Atrial fibrillation interrupted by a paroxysm of ventricular tachycardia. In the top strip, there is a wide-beat tachycardia that might be ventricular or junctional with aberrancy. In the bottom strip there is progressive fusion between the impulses from the ventricular tachycardia and those conducted down from the fibrillating atria. The very rapid rate of the narrow beats also rules out any possibility of rate-dependent aberrancy as an explanation for the wide beats. (At the right-hand end of the bottom strip the lead changes to avr.)

A

B

Atrial Fibrillation with Rate-Dependent Bundle-Branch Block

Atrial fibrillation with fixed bundle-branch block is no problem. As in Fig. 9-18 there are the typical wide QRS complexes appearing irregularly, without P waves. The QRS complexes do not change even when the rate varies.

Rate-dependent bundle-branch block can produce patterns that might be confused with paroxysms of ventricular tachycardia, but the distinction is simple. In Fig. 9-19 there are periods of wide-beat tachycardia interrupted by occasional normally conducted beats. In the pauses there are obvious "f" waves. The wide-beat rhythm is totally irregular, with some R-R intervals twice as wide as others. The rate in ventricular tachycardia can vary a little, but never that much. Whenever the rate slows below a certain point, the QRS is normal. This is obviously rate-dependent bundle-branch block and not ventricular tachycardia.

Clinical note: When you're considering the possibility of rate-dependent bundle-branch block, slow the ventricular rate by carotid massage or adenosine. You'll have the answer in seconds.

FIGURE 9-18
Stable right bundle-branch block with atrial fibrillation. Note the characteristic wide variation in R-R as in any atrial fibrillation.

FIGURE 9-19
Atrial fibrillation with rate-dependent bundle-branch block. Whenever the rate slows, as in the bottom strip, the QRS narrows. Note also the very wide variation in R-R intervals, characteristic of conduction from fibrillating atria.

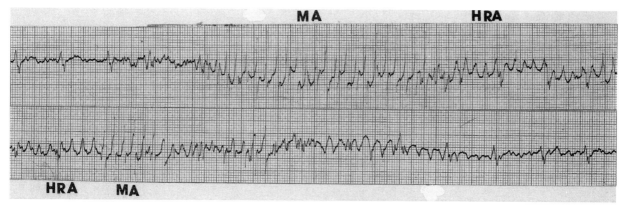

FIGURE 9-20
Intra-atrial recording of atrial fibrillation. Note the progressive enlargement of the "F" waves as the electrode moves through the superior vena cava and into the right atrium. Complexes arising in the high right atrium (HRA) are large and irregularly "saw-toothed"; complexes arising in the midatrium (MA) are huge, narrow spikes.

What Fibrillary Waves Look Like Inside the Atria

When you're localizing a transvenous pacemaker electrocardiographically, you have to know what fibrillary waves look like inside the atria. Figure 9-20 records the change from ordinary surface "f" waves to the giant "spiky" inscriptions recorded when the electrode is in the right atrium. The atrial deflections are huge, much larger than the ventricular complexes, and they're sharp and narrow. MA refers to atrial impulses recorded from the mid-right atrium. HRA refers to impulses recorded when the electrode was withdrawn to the high right atrium at the junction with the superior vena cava.

10 | Atrial Flutter

The salient point to pin in your memory about atrial flutter is that the atrial rhythm is absolutely regular. Atrial flutter is a remarkable mechanism: The complexes it produces are precise in timing and shape within a hundredth of a millimeter and a hundredth of a second. If there is the slightest variation in the atrial complexes, the rhythm isn't flutter.

You make the diagnosis of atrial flutter by recognizing flutter waves in the ECG. (It's alleged that you can recognize flutter waves in the jugular venous pulse, but this is so rare that it's no more than a pious hope. You can probably see jugular flutter waves only about one time out of ten.)

The first thing you notice about typical flutter waves is that there's no flat, isoelectric period between them. The end of one wave is the beginning of the next; this produces the classic "saw-toothed" configuration (Fig. 10-1). It also reflects the continuous atrial activity of flutter. The atrial rate here is 300; with the usual 2:1 conduction, the ventricular rate is 150. In Fig. 10-2 the flutter rate is much slower — about 188. The precise reproduction and timing of each flutter wave is obvious. In the bottom strip carotid sinus pressure was applied so that the flutter waves are isolated, with only two ventricular responses in the whole strip. Note also the different appearance of flutter waves in the different leads.

Figure 10-3 is another example of 2:1 flutter. One negative "sawtooth" is about 0.16 seconds ahead of the QRS, while the other comes just after the QRS (arrows). Place the tips of your calipers on these two negative deflections and you'll see that they march out perfectly with a rate of 215.

In Fig. 10-4 you see an important variant in flutter. The ratio of conduction changes from 2:1 to 3:1 and 4:1 in various parts of the strip. The ventricular response is therefore completely irregular, and at the bedside it couldn't be distinguished from atrial fibrillation.

FIGURE 10-1
Typical flutter waves in
the limb leads. Note how
prominent the flutter
waves are in II, III, and
avf, while you can't see
them in I and avl.

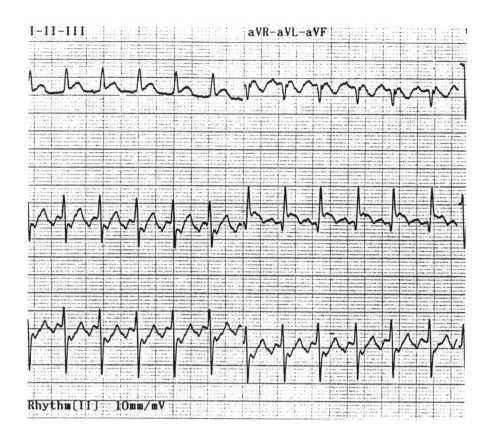

One-third of all cases of atrial flutter will manifest changing ratios of conduction to the ventricles with an irregular ventricular rhythm. (A few years ago while I was lecturing on this topic, a physician stood up and maintained with some heat that if the ratio of conduction changes, "you have to call it fibrillation!" Nothing could be further from the truth. The accident of conduction down the AV node has nothing to do with what's happening in the atria.)

Where do you see flutter waves? They tend to be isolated. Usually you see them in only one lead system — II, III, and avf as a rule. In Fig. 10-5 the flutter waves are obvious in II, III, and avf, but you'd have a hard time recognizing them anywhere else. There's a small "glitch" just after the peak of the T in these leads that represents the nonconducted flutter wave; if you look closely you can see the same deflection in V4, 5, and 6.

Sometimes flutter waves are visible in only one lead. Figure 10-6 is a dramatic example of this phenomenon. There are large, unmistakable flutter waves in V1, but you can't find anything in the other leads that you could positively identify as a flutter wave. In the limb leads, there's not a clue.

FIGURE 10-2
Relatively slow flutter
waves in the limb leads.
The period of carotid sinus
pressure in lead III gives
you a chance to see the isolated flutter waves. Note
the mathematical regular-
ity.

FIGURE 10-3
2:1 flutter.

FIGURE 10-4
Flutter with varying ratios
of conduction to the ven-
tricles. Note grossly irregular ventricular rhythm.

The ECG tracing contains the following text annotations:

Atrial flutter, ventricular rate 86, atrial rate 250
1 VPC, except for arrhythmia, tracing is not outside normal
limits.

BRENDAN PHIBBS, MD 1/19/93im

Rhythm[II] 10mm/mV

Lead labels at top: I-II-III, aVR-aVL-aVF, V1-V2-V3, V4-V5-V6

FIGURE 10-5
Prominent flutter waves in II, III, and avf. The flutter waves are practically invisible in the other leads. (You can see tiny deflections in V4–6.)

Two Tips for Identifying Flutter Waves

Figure 10-7 illustrates a typical 2:1 flutter. Note two characteristics of the flutter waves:

1. The alternate flutter wave intersects the QRS *above* the baseline. When you see this consistently through a strip, you're dealing with flutter: Flutter waves are the only atrial complexes that do this.

2. You can draw an imaginary line from the top of the flutter wave just before the QRS down through the ventricular complex and see the flutter wave emerge on the other side.

Watch for these two unique characteristics of flutter waves.

Since the diagnosis of flutter rests on your visual recognition of flutter waves, here are some examples of the different forms they can take.

In Fig. 10-8, the flutter waves are really hard to see. At the right side of the tracing you can see very small, perfect "spikes" as indicated by the arrows. They're most obvious when the ratio shifts to 3:1. In the pause between QRS complexes the tiny flutter waves are clearly visible, with a rate of 300. Once you've identified them you can follow them all the way through the tracing with a pair of calipers.

FIGURE 10-6
Isolated flutter waves in V1 only. They're absolutely invisible everywhere else. Be sure to look at all leads before you rule out flutter!

FIGURE 10-7
A simple trick for recognizing flutter waves is to follow a flutter wave through the QRS complex.

FIGURE 10-8
Tiny but definite flutter waves (arrows) that become really visible only when the ratio of conduction shifts.

FIGURE 10-9
Comparison of flutter waves in inferior leads (II, III, avf) and V1. In V1, flutter waves often appear as small, discrete atrial complexes, resembling rapidly inscribed P waves. In this case the atrial rate would reveal the diagnosis even if you couldn't see the obvious flutter waves in the inferior leads.

Figure 10-9 illustrates another variation. You see typical flutter waves in II, III, and avf, but if you look at V1 you see what flutter waves usually look like in the right precordium. They're commonly small, discrete, upright waves not at all like the saw-toothed waves you see in the limb leads.

If you look at the examples so far you can see that the atrial rate in flutter can range from as high as 300 down to 210 or 215. In the adult heart the atrial rate will practically never exceed 300.

Vagal Stimulation in the Diagnosis of Flutter

Sometimes it's absolutely impossible to diagnose flutter until you cause a block in the AV node that lets you see the isolated flutter waves. Figure 10-10 is an excellent example. Looking at the right-hand side of the strip only, you couldn't possibly make the diagnosis. Carotid sinus stimulation blocked transmission through the AV node and made the flutter obvious.

Figures 10-11, 10-12, and 10-13 are examples of obscure flutter unmasked by carotid sinus stimulation. Now that adenosine is available, temporary blockade of the AV node is even easier and safer. Use this maneuver whenever you see a baffling supraventricular rhythm like the ones illustrated here.

FIGURE 10-10
Unmasking of atrial flutter by carotid sinus stimulation. It would not be possible to make a diagnosis from the right-hand part of the strip.

FIGURE 10-11
Unmasking of atrial flutter by carotid sinus stimulation. The flutter waves are tiny (arrows) but absolutely regular. Without AV nodal blockade, diagnosis would be impossible.

FIGURE 10-12
Unmasking of atrial flutter by carotid sinus stimulation. The left side of the strip looks remarkably like a normal sinus rhythm! (Thank your resident deity for adenosine in cases like this.)

FIGURE 10-13
A baffling arrhythmia that was unmasked only by carotid sinus stimulation while V3-R was being recorded. *Always* use AV nodal blockade, and *always* record numerous different leads when tracking down obscure flutter.

To diagnose block in the presence of atrial flutter, you need only to substitute flutter waves for sinus P waves and the problem becomes simple. In Fig. 10-14 you see a slow, regular ventricular rhythm with a rate of 43. Now look carefully at the flutter waves ahead of each QRS. *Note that there's a changing relation of flutter wave to QRS.* That's analogous to seeing a changing P-R when the sinus node is discharging. Despite the changing flutter-R relation, the ventricular rhythm is absolutely regular.

FIGURE 10-14
Complete AV nodal block in the presence of flutter. Instead of a changing P-R relation, look for a changing flutter-R in the presence of a regular ventricular rhythm to establish the diagnosis of dissociation.

The diagnosis is therefore complete AV dissociation. The ventricular rhythm arises in the AV junction, and the flutter waves never penetrate to the ventricles. Since the ventricular rate is 43, all the criteria for complete heart block are present.

In Fig. 10-15 there is obviously a high degree of block, but it's not complete. The ventricular rhythm is irregular, and if you look closely there are minute changes in the relation of flutter waves to QRS complexes.

Figure 10-16 is an example of complete block in the presence of atrial flutter. There are two idioventricular foci discharging at different rates. The ventricular rhythm is regular for short periods (the first four beats on the top strip and the last four on the right-hand side of the bottom strip). During these periods of regular ventricular firing, the relation of flutter wave to QRS changes in a totally random manner. There is therefore complete heart block with two idioventricular pacemakers discharging.

FIGURE 10-15
High degree of AV nodal block in the presence of atrial flutter. The changing R-R interval tells you the block probably isn't complete.

FIGURE 10-16
Complete AV block in the presence of atrial flutter. Multiple idioventricular pacemakers.

FIGURE 10-17
Atrial flutter with complete AV block. Note the changing flutter-R relationship with the regular slow ventricular rhythm.

Figure 10-17 is an example of simple complete block with a ventricular rate of 26. Look carefully at the flutter-QRS relation and you'll see that it changes throughout the strip, thus confirming complete AV dissociation.

Wenckebach Block in the Presence of Atrial Flutter

In Fig. 10-18 there is a definite paired, or "bigeminal," rhythm with obvious flutter waves. The diagram below explains what's happening. In ordinary 2:1 flutter, one flutter wave is conducted and one isn't. The flutter wave that isn't conducted doesn't penetrate the AV node at all. In other words, in flutter there is always one level of block between the atria and the AV node. Many times there will be some kind of block to the impulse that does go down the AV node, thus there's a second level of block.

The trick to recognizing this is to ignore the alternate flutter waves that don't penetrate the AV node at all and concentrate on the ones that do. In other words, look for a pattern of block on the alternate flutter wave, as illustrated in Fig. 10-18. Ignore the nonconducted flutter waves and look at the alternate ones that penetrate the AV node. Here there's an absolutely regular pattern of progressive prolongation of flutter-QRS

FIGURE 10-18
Two-level block with atrial flutter. Wenckebach block to the alternate flutter impulses.

until the third alternate flutter wave is blocked. Like any 3:2 block, this gives a paired, or "bigeminal," rhythm.

1:1 Flutter and How to Avoid It

It's fortunate that every flutter wave doesn't reach the ventricles: The heart would usually race itself to death if they did. There are two conditions when 1:1 flutter can occur.

1-A Drugs

Quinidine and procaine amide can both produce 1:1 flutter — especially quinidine. There are two reasons for this:

1. Both quinidine and procaine amide are mildly vagolytic: By enhancing sympathetic drive, they accelerate conduction through the AV node. This is actually a minor effect.

2. Both drugs slow the flutter rate in the atria. A flutter that's been firing at 300 may slow to 210–215. At this rate it's possible for every wave to penetrate the AV node and pull the ventricular rate up to the atrial rate. The results may be catastrophic.

Rule: Never give a 1-A drug for flutter until there's adequate blockade of the AV node by digitalis or other drugs to prevent 1:1 conduction.

Figure 10-19 is an example of 1:1 flutter caused by administration of

FIGURE 10-19
1:1 atrial flutter caused by administration of quinidine without digitalis or other source of AV nodal blockade.

I-II-III　　　aVR-aVL-aVF　　　V1-V2-V3　　　V4-V5-V6

Rhythm (II) 10mm/mV

quinidine without digitalis. Atrial and ventricular rates are both 250. At this point, of course, the patient was critical, and only rapid AV nodal blockade saved his life.

Exercise

The patient who complains to you about pounding of the heart during exercise may be describing this phenomenon.

In Fig. 10-20 you see what happened during a treadmill test. From a sinus rate of 118 the patient suddenly went into a very rapid tachycardia with a rate of 215. There was no way of knowing what this rhythm was until there was transient slowing as a result of carotid sinus stimulation

FIGURE 10-20
Tracing recorded during treadmill exercise. After three sinus beats a tachycardia appears that settles down to a steady rate of 215.

FIGURE 10-21
With carotid sinus stimulation and slowing of the rate, obvious flutter waves can be seen (F). The rate of the flutter waves is exactly the same as the ventricular rate: 215. This is exercise-induced 1:1 flutter.

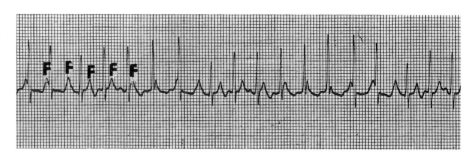

(Fig. 10-21). Here you can clearly see flutter waves (F). If you measure the flutter rate you'll see that it's 215 — exactly the same as the ventricular rate on the right-hand side of the tracing. This is *exercise-induced 1:1 flutter.* The surge of catecholamines that accompanies exercise enhances AV conduction and allows every flutter wave to reach the ventricles. Keep this possibility in mind when people tell you they "feel as if their heart is racing" during tennis or bicycling!

Self-Assessment II

FIGURE II-1

1. Conduction defect? Degree? Where localized?

FIGURE II-2

2. Lead V1. Diagnosis?

FIGURE II-3

3. Complete description? The patient is taking unknown "heart medicine." Probable diagnosis?

FIGURE II-4

4. Complete description? Significance of wide beats? Treatment, if any?

FIGURE II-5

5. Conduction defect? Can you localize it? Possibilities and significance?

FIGURE II-6

6. Changing rhythm. Diagnosis?

FIGURE II-7

7. Rapid irregular ventricular rhythm. Diagnosis?

FIGURE II-8

8. Conduction defect? Possible sites? Significance? Treatment, if any?

FIGURE II-9   9. Changing rate and rhythm, changing QRS width. Cause? Significance?

FIGURE II-10   10. Rhythm? Mechanism(s)?

FIGURE II-11   11. Rhythm?

FIGURE II-12   12. Rhythm? State of AV conduction?

FIGURE II-13   13. Grossly irregular rhythm. Diagnosis?

FIGURE II-14   14. Basic rhythm. Cause of pauses?

FIGURE II-15

15. You have a pacing wire in the right atrium, pacing at a rate of 77. The following pattern appears. Significance? Treatment, if any?

FIGURE II-16

16. The patient is distressed but the pulse is regular, rate 115. What's really going on? How can you tell?

FIGURE II-17

17. Irregular irregularity of the pulse. Cause?

FIGURE II-18

18. Wide beats, narrow beats, blocked P waves. What's happening and where?

FIGURE II-19

19. State of AV conduction? Block or no block? What's going on during the first seven beats and what does it mean?

FIGURE II-20

20. Almost-regular rate with occasional pauses. Diagnosis? Anatomic site of problem?

Answers

1. Complete AV block, localized in the AV node. Note all the criteria for complete block.
2. Coarse atrial fibrillation. Even though the fibrillary waves are large and regular for short periods, they're much too fast for flutter and their rate and shape change if you look closely. Atrial rate in flutter will never be faster than 300 in the adult heart.
3. Atrial fibrillation with a high degree of heart block. The conducted beats are slightly irregular, indicating that the block isn't complete. Reentrant VPCs are present. Digitalis toxicity!
4. Atrial fibrillation interrupted by runs of accelerated idioventricular rhythm. This is benign and should cause the cardiologist only to look for long pauses in conduction that lead to the escape of the ventricular focus.
5. 2:1 AV block with bundle-branch block. The block could be localized in the AV node or in the other bundle branch, which would make it a variant of Type II block. You can't make the distinction from this tracing alone.
6. Paroxysms of atrial flutter with two sinus beats.
7. Atrial flutter. Note the typical "saw-toothed" atrial complexes in the wider R-R intervals in the middle of the strip.

8. Complete AV block. The wide complexes of the dissociated ventricular rhythm raise two possibilities: This could be AV nodal block with a junctional rhythm and bundle-branch block *or* it could be bilateral bundle-branch block with an idioventricular rhythm — much more serious!

9. Mobitz-II block. Fixed P-R in two or more consecutive beats before the blocked P, same P-R after the blocked P as before, bundle-branch block. Typical. Additional feature: rate-dependent bundle-branch block. Pacemaker!

10. Atrial fibrillation, bundle-branch block, runs of junctional tachycardia producing the regular wide-beat rhythm. Occasional ventricular ectopic beats.

11. Again, very coarse flutter or flutter-fibrillation. Don't confuse this with true flutter. The changing morphology of the atrial complexes is the tip-off.

12. Atrial fibrillation with complete AV nodal block.

13. Paroxysms of atrial flutter with junctional rhythm between paroxysms.

14. Tricky. Atrial flutter with runs of completely dissociated junctional rhythm. Note regular ventricular rhythm with totally random relation of flutter waves to QRS — this is the same as a regular ventricular rhythm with a changing P-R: It equals dissociation. High degree of AV block, but the ventricular rate is too rapid to permit diagnosis of complete AV block. (Tracing courtesy of Dr. Frank Marcus.)

15. Mobitz-II block revealed during atrial pacing. Bundle-branch block with all the criteria for Mobitz-II block. Pacemaker!

16. 2:1 atrial flutter. Note typical "saw-teeth" between ventricular complexes.

17. Wenckebach block. Three conducted beats with extreme prolongation of the last P-R: The blocked P is half-hidden in the last QRS of the cycle. The QRS following the very prolonged P-R may in fact be a junctional escape beat so that there would be two nonconducted P waves in each cycle.

18. V1. The first two beats show a typical Wenckebach progression with block of the third P wave. Right bundle-branch block is present: The pause after the blocked P reveals that the bundle-branch block is rate-dependent. The fourth P wave is also blocked, and Wenckebach periods resume on the right-hand side of the strip. Diagnosis: AV nodal block with rate-dependent bundle-branch block.

19. The first, second, fourth, and fifth beats in the top strip and the first two beats in the bottom strip are clearly dissociated from the sinus P waves. Beat 3 in the top strip and the last three beats in the bottom strip are sinus beats. Thus there is a basic sinus rhythm with periods

of dissociation caused by the discharge of an idioventricular pacemaker. Is block present? Of course not, the sinus beats tell you that! *The reason for the intermittent dissociation is the slow sinus rate — about 42 — which permits "escape" of the idioventricular focus.* Remember the last commandment in the diagnosis of complete heart block: "enough atrial impulses to probe all aspects of diastole."

20. Long Wenckebach runs with very gradual prolongation of P-R. The large deflection following the QRS is a P wave, and you can see it moving minutely closer to the preceding QRS with each beat until one P wave is finally blocked.

11

Preexcitation

Preexcitation pathways, or "bypass tracts," are strands of conducting tissue that have the capacity to bypass part or all of the AV conducting system. Let's start with two general statements:

1. Bypass tracts can conduct very rapidly — over 300 beats per minute in many cases.
2. Bypass tracts have no innervation. They are not affected by the sympathetic or parasympathetic systems or by drugs that work through those systems.

There are three general classes of bypass tracts; if you understand how they're connected you can reason out the ECG configuration with each.

Wolff-Parkinson-White (WPW) Conduction

This was the first type of bypass tract to be described anatomically and electrocardiographically.

A bypass tract called the Kent bundle is located out in the AV groove, relatively far from the AV node (Fig. 11-1). The bypass tract completely "short-circuits" the AV node; since bypass tissue conducts rapidly, the P-R is short — less than 0.12 seconds in the adult heart. Thus the short P-R interval is the first element in recognition of WPW preexcitation.

The bypass tract inserts in the bundle-branch system below the bifurcation of the bundle branches. This eccentric activation causes a deformity, or "slurring," of the initial part of the QRS as part of the impulse moves backward up toward the common bundle while the rest moves normally forward (Fig. 11-1). This combination of events produces the typical slurred R wave or "delta-R" first described in WPW conduction. The slurring can also be a negative deflection, depending on what lead you're looking at, so the best term is *delta wave*.

FIGURE 11-1
Anatomy of a Wolff-
Parkinson-White bypass
tract.

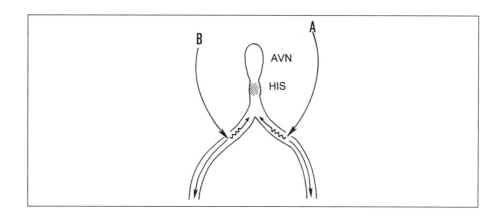

FIGURE 11-2
Typical WPW preexcita-
tion. Arrow indicates delta
wave.

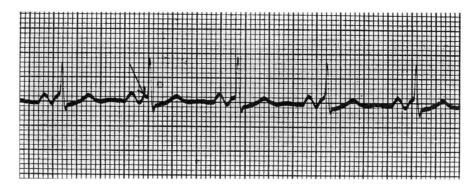

The delta wave is a slowly inscribed deflection; it reflects the relatively slow retrograde force moving back up toward the common bundle. Often this wave collides with the normal antegrade impulse coming down through the AV node so that there's a kind of fusion. The delta wave may be larger or smaller, depending on where the fusion takes place. If the retrograde impulse travels all the way to the common bundle and "over the top" into the other side, the deflection is called the "full" preexcitation pattern.

Figure 11-2 is a typical example of WPW preexcitation. The short P-R and the delta wave are obvious, but from this strip alone you couldn't localize the preexcitation.

The first attempt at anatomic localization of a bypass tract was relatively simple. If the bypass tract inserts in the *left* bundle, V1 will look like *right* bundle-branch block, except that the QRS will usually be narrower. There will be a typical delta-R wave leading into a broad R (Fig. 11-3). This was called Type A WPW for the rather naive reason that V1 looks like an "A." (The reason that preexciting into the left bundle pro-

FIGURE 11-3
Type A WPW. The wide, slurred initial part of the R wave is obvious across the precordial leads and in leads II, III, and avf.

duces a right bundle-branch block pattern is elementary. When right bundle-branch block is present, the order of activation is first left ventricle then right ventricle. When the left bundle is preexcited, of course, the same sequence follows: left ventricle first, right ventricle second.)

If the Kent bundle attaches to the right bundle, V1 will look like left bundle-branch block. The delta wave will be directed downward. The QRS won't usually be as wide as in left bundle-branch block, but it will consist of a broad S wave (Fig. 11-4). This is called Type B WPW.

This elementary differentiation still has some validity. Modern studies have shown that when Type A is present, the bypass tract often lies in the left posteroseptal area, whereas when Type B is present, the connection lies anteriorly and rightward.

With the help of mapping techniques it has become clear that the picture is much more complicated than everyone thought. In fact at least ten possible sites for atrioventricular bypass tracts have been identified, but the common feature in all is the short P-R interval with deformity of the first part of the QRS. At least 90% of the cases you will see will fit into the Type A or Type B category, and that's about as far as the clinical electrocardiographer needs to go. There have been attempts to localize the bypass tract more precisely by the orientation of the delta force, but they are relevant only if ablation is contemplated, at which point precise intracardiac mapping is necessary in any case. What the clinical electrocardiographer needs to recognize is preexcitation per se.

Lown-Ganong-Levine (LGL) Preexcitation

This may in fact be the most common form of preexcitation. There's a short P-R interval with a *normal* QRS. How can this happen? Consider Fig. 11-5A and B.

FIGURE 11-4
Type B WPW. Note the
wide, downward deflec-
tion in V1 with slurring of
the initial part of the complex. The slurring is the
delta wave, here seen as a
negative deflection. The
delta wave is clearly visible in leads I and II, V3–6.

Remember that you can have a normal QRS only if the impulse comes
from above, down the normal bundle-branch tract. In LGL preexcitation
that's exactly what happens. A special kind of bypass tract, called a
James fiber (after Thomas James, the discoverer), connects the atria to
the His bundle. There's a short P-R because the AV node has been by-
passed, but conduction down through the ventricles is normal. The
whole diagnosis depends on recognizing the short P-R interval (Fig. 11-
5B). That's why the magic minimum number of 0.12 seconds for normal
AV conduction has to be burned into the electrocardiographer's brain.
Some recent investigators have suggested that a short P-R may be simply a normal variant, but a P-R like the one in Fig. 11-5B cannot be the
result of anything but LGL preexcitation — always assuming you've
made sure those are normal sinus P waves and have thus ruled out a
junctional rhythm.

FIGURE 11-5

LGL type of preexcitation. (A) The bypass tract, probably a James fiber, connects the atria to the His bundle. The activating impulse follows a normal course down through the bundle-branch system. As a result, there is a short P-R interval and the QRS is normal. (B) The P-R is about 0.09 seconds, and the QRS is 0.08 seconds.

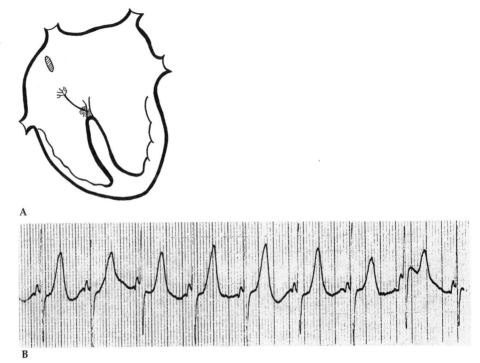

A

B

Mahaim Fiber Preexcitation

Figure 11-6 illustrates another type of preexcitation, caused by small "jump" or "short-circuit" fibers described by Mahaim. They may connect the AV node or the His bundle directly to the bundle-branch system. In either case there will be a typical delta wave and usually some degree of P-R shortening. If a Mahaim fiber originates low in the His, however, the P-R may be within the limits of normal, and the only hint of preexcitation will be the delta wave. In this case you could only suspect preexcitation but you couldn't prove it from the surface ECG.

FIGURE 11-6

Mahaim fibers. As indicated, these are usually short tracts that can lead from the AV node or the His bundle to some part of the bundle-branch system.

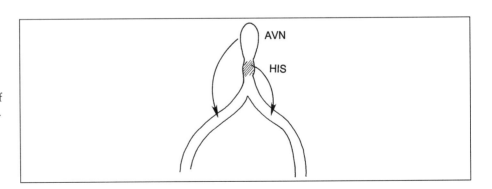

Why is Preexcitation Important?

Preexcitation and Arrhythmias

With a bypass tract there is a perfect setup for a "circus" movement. An impulse can come down the bypass tract and back up the AV node, around and around in a self-perpetuating circuit. It can also go the other way around, down the AV node and back up the bypass tract (Fig. 11-7A and B). In either case, there will be a *paroxysmal supraventricular tachycardia.* Patients with bypass tracts may have recurrent paroxysms of supraventricular tachycardia because they have the anatomic setup for it.

If there is WPW preexcitation, you can tell which way the impulse is traveling by looking at the ECG. If the impulse is coming down the bypass tract, there will be a typical deformed QRS with a delta wave (Fig. 11-8). If the impulse comes down the AV node, the QRS will be normal. Just by looking at the ECG during the tachycardia, you couldn't tell that there was a bypass tract (Fig. 11-9).

With the LGL type of preexcitation, the QRS complexes are normal, and the tachycardia will look like any other paroxysmal supraventricular tachycardia.

Moral: When a patient has recurrent paroxysmal tachycardia, you have to consider preexcitation whether the QRS complexes show a "delta R" or not.

Bypass Tracts with Atrial Fibrillation

(This book is primarily about diagnosis, not treatment, but in this specific setting, the two are so closely intertwined that they have to be considered together.)

FIGURE 11-7
Mechanisms of paroxysmal tachycardia. (A) Antidromic bypass tract. Circuit is down the bypass tract and back through the AV node. The QRS will be abnormal with a typical delta wave. (B) Orthodromic bypass tract. Circuit is down the AV node and back through the bypass tract. The QRS will be normal.

The slow conduction of the AV is often lifesaving. That's especially true in atrial fibrillation, as we pointed out in Chap. 9. The AV node protects the ventricles from being bombarded 425 times a minute by the impulses from the fibrillating atria. When there's a bypass tract, that protection is weakened. The bypass tract can conduct very rapidly, up to 300 times a minute. The heart would race itself to death if this happened for very long. The only reason it doesn't is that some impulses come down the AV node and make the ventricular tissues refractory to the impulses from the bypass tract. Thus there is a kind of "competition" between the AV node and the bypass tract: The AV node acts as a "brake" on the bypass tract and keeps it from driving the ventricles into a disaster (Fig. 11-10).

How can you tell there's preexcitation when the patient is fibrillating? After all, there are no P waves to measure from. There are two clues. First, there may be typical delta waves with deformed QRS complexes (Fig. 11-11). Second, you can get a pretty good idea from the rate. *Bypass tracts conduct rapidly.* They conduct faster than the AV node could possibly conduct.

1. If you see R-R intervals equal to a rate of 300 (one large square apart), you can be certain there's a bypass tract.

2. If you see R-R intervals equal to a rate of 280 or more, you can make the diagnosis of a bypass tract with about 99% confidence.

FIGURE 11-9

Paroxysmal tachycardia in a patient with Type B WPW. The activating impulse is coming down the AV node, producing a normal QRS. Just by looking at this tracing, you couldn't tell there was a bypass tract.

3. If you see many R-R intervals equal to a rate of over 250, you should be very suspicious of a bypass tract (Figs. 11-11 and 11-12).

Detecting a bypass tract in the presence of atrial fibrillation can be of life-and-death importance. Why? Simple. The first drug you think of when you treat atrial fibrillation is digitalis. Digitalis slows conduction through the AV node but has no effect on bypass tracts. If you depress AV nodal conduction with digitalis, you remove the "brake," and the bypass tract can run wild. The heart rate can race into a catastrophe.

The same thing is true of verapamil, beta-blocking drugs, and many calcium-blocking drugs. They depress the AV node without affecting the bypass tract. With any of these drugs the resulting rapid rate can produce congestive heart failure or a fatal arrhythmia.

The only safe drugs to use in this setting are quinidine and procaine amide. They both depress conduction through the bypass tract. They are the only safe drugs that do. The 1-C drugs encainide and flecainide are excellent for depressing bypass-tract conduction, but they're so dangerous that encainide isn't even on the market anymore. Flecainide could be used in an otherwise healthy patient, but it's excessively dangerous if there's any depression of AV function.

FIGURE 11-10
Atrial fibrillation in the presence of a bypass tract. Note dual pathways from atria to ventricles, one down the AV nodal path and one down the bypass tract. The impulses that come down the AV node will make the conducting tissues refractory to some of the impulses from the bypass tract. Thus the AV node acts as a brake on the bypass tract, which could otherwise drive the heart at a rate that might well be fatal. Drugs like digitalis and verapamil that depress conduction through the AV node without affecting the bypass tract can be lethal in this situation.

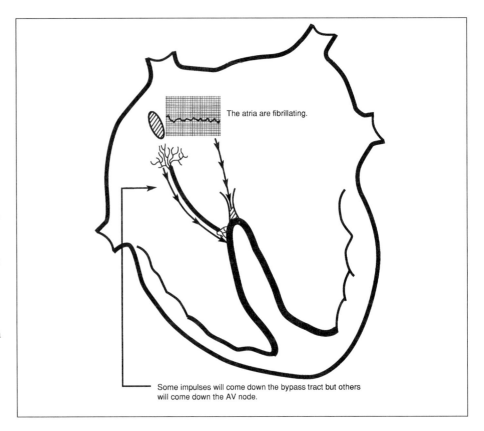

The atria are fibrillating.

Some impulses will come down the bypass tract but others will come down the AV node.

Moral: Whenever you confront a new case of atrial fibrillation, look for the signs of preexcitation — the "delta R" or the rapid rate (or both). If there is any suspicion of preexcitation, don't use digitalis or verapamil until you have carried out a simple test that will tell you with 100% accuracy whether preexcitation is present or not.

Test? What test? This test can be carried out in any emergency room or clinic where there's an ECG machine. It's based on the fact that bypass tracts have no nerve supply. If you stimulate the vagus you may slow conduction through the AV node but you won't affect the bypass tract.

1. Stimulate the vagus by carotid massage. If the rate slows, there's no bypass tract. If the rate speeds, a bypass tract is present. Think about it for a moment and you'll see how it works.

2. If carotid sinus stimulation is ineffective, administer adenosine. Adenosine slows AV nodal conduction but has no effect on bypass tissue. Use the same logic as above.

FIGURE 11-11
Atrial fibrillation with Type A WPW. Besides the wide, slurred QRS complexes, the preexcitation is obvious in the rate. Note the R-R interval indicated by an arrow; it's equivalent to a rate of 300.

In either case be sure to keep a rhythm strip running all the time and watch for changes in rate.

Note: Administration of adenosine during atrial fibrillation to rule out a bypass tract is an excellent and very specific maneuver, but it's not harmless. During the six seconds or so of AV nodal blockade that is induced by adenosine, the bypass tract can drive the ventricles into fibrillation; this has already been recorded in two case reports when the patients were only saved by prompt defibrillation. **When administering adenosine to rule out preexcitation during atrial fibrillation always have a defibrillator on standby!**

Bypass Tracts and "Artificial" QRS Deformity
The odd initial force, or delta wave, can show up in some leads as a negative deflection, or Q wave. People with perfectly normal hearts may be

FIGURE 11-12
Examples of atrial fibrillation with preexcitation. The QRS complexes are normal, but the very rapid rate is the clue. Many R-R intervals are equivalent to rates over 250, which makes preexcitation probable. LGL preexcitation was in fact present in these cases.

FIGURE 11-13
"Pathologic" Q waves in avf are really upside-down delta waves. The clue is the presence of obvious delta waves in other leads.

told they've had a myocardial infarct when all they have is preexcitation (Figs. 11-13 and 11-14).

The bypass tract may attach so far down the bundle branch that it produces a full-blown bundle-branch block pattern (Fig. 11-15).

What do you do if you find preexcitation in a routine ECG? Another simple answer. If the patient is asymptomatic you don't do anything. You inform the patient that this congenital "short circuit" is present because the knowledge might be helpful if tachycardia or fibrillation appeared. Beyond that you do nothing. You don't frighten the patient,

FIGURE 11-14
"Pathologic" Q wave in avl. (This is another one of those leads you'll learn about in Chap. 17, Myocardial Infarction.) The obvious delta R waves in II, III, and avf reveal that this supposed Q wave is simply an inverted delta wave.

FIGURE 11-15
Intermittent WPW preexcitation producing a pattern like bundle-branch block. The obvious clue is the short P-R interval of the wide beats. The bypass tract must insert far down the bundle branch to produce this kind of pattern.

because the chances of a serious complication are 1:40,000 in an otherwise normal individual! (Some enthusiasts recently recommended that all patients with preexcitation undergo exhaustive invasive testing. They were roundly rebuked by competent authorities, and certainly there are no data to support such an approach. Don't subject patients to stress, fear, pain, and expense for an anomaly that will probably never mean a thing.) Figures 11-16 through 11-20 are typical examples of preexcitation in various settings.

FIGURE 11-16
Intermittent WPW. The wide QRS complexes represent WPW preexcitation; the narrow beats with inverted P waves are actually ectopic atrial beats with normal conduction.

FIGURE 11-17
Intermittent WPW with occasional normally conducted beats. This would be very easy to confuse with bundle-branch block, but the short P-R is the clue to the diagnosis, as well as the appearance of occasional normally conducted beats.

FIGURE 11-18
Normal sinus rhythm interrupted by two WPW beats.

FIGURE 11-19
Atrial fibrillation with WPW. Note the short runs of beats with a rate approximating 300 as well as the wide, deformed QRS complexes.

FIGURE 11-20
LGL preexcitation with ventricular ectopic beats.

Note that in Figs. 11-15, 11-16, 11-17, 11-18, and 11-20 the preexcitation is intermittent. I find that this observation often comes as a surprise to physicians-in-training, but in fact, intermittent preexcitation is very common. Moral: Whenever you see mixtures of wide and narrow QRS complexes, look carefully at the P-R of the assorted beats to see if the wide complexes represent preexcitation!

12 | Fascicular Beats and Fascicular Tachycardia

For years electrocardiographers were puzzled by the problem of the "narrow VPC." Look at the ectopic beat in Fig. 12-1. It looks like a VPC in every respect except that it's too narrow to qualify. This ectopic beat is about 0.10 to 0.11 seconds wide, whereas a real VPC should always be at least 0.12 seconds wide. Note the extreme left axis of the same ectopic beat: It's about –60°.

The first thing everybody noticed about these "narrow VPCs" was that all had an extreme left or right axis. Another feature quickly became apparent; it's illustrated in Figs. 12-2 and 12-3. In each of these tracings the ectopic beat has an extreme right axis — about +120° to

FIGURE 12-1
Note the slightly narrow VPC with an extreme left axis. For years these beats were a puzzle.

FIGURE 12-2

Note the "narrow" ectopic beats (arrows). They are not preceded by P waves and they have a completely different QRST shape from the sinus beats, but they're not as wide as ordinary VPCs. They have an extreme right axis and an incomplete right bundle-branch block configuration in V1.

+130°. If you look at V1 in each tracing you'll notice one or more ectopic beats with an incomplete right bundle-branch block pattern. One explanation for these odd beats was that they were junctional beats that followed a different course through the ventricles because of their "off-center" origin.

Electrophysiologic studies, however, have demonstrated that at least in many cases, these beats arise in a branch of the left bundle branch. Remember that the functional elements of the left bundle are called "fascicles." Ectopic beats can originate in these fascicles. Cells high in the fascicles of the bundle-branch system may take on the characteristics of pacemaker cells and start generating beats. Since these beats are traveling down the specialized conducting cells of the bundle branches at 4 m/sec., they move faster than ventricular ectopic beats moving "backward" through the subendocardium. That's why they're narrow.

A beat that arises in the posterior fascicle will naturally have an extreme left axis, because that's where the posterior fascicle conducts. Anterior fascicular beats will have an extreme right axis for the same reason. In V1 these beats will show a pattern of right bundle-branch delay with an R-R' configuration, because the fascicular beat has to fight its way backward up the left bundle branch and across and down the right bundle branch (Fig. 12-4).

For a long time this was nothing more than a curiosity, interesting only to investigators. Then observers began to notice tachycardias like the ones shown in Figs. 12-5 and 12-6. These are wide-beat tachycardias with all the ECG characteristics of paroxysmal ventricular tachycardia.

FIGURE 12-3
Same phenomenon. Ectopic beats about 0.09 seconds wide, extreme right axis, incomplete right bundle-branch block pattern in V1.

However, the ventricular complexes show a right bundle-branch block configuration with an extreme left axis. This tachycardia is clinically different from any other ventricular tachycardia. It usually appears in relatively young, otherwise healthy individuals and it never causes catastrophic symptoms — that is, the patient doesn't collapse or go into shock. The usual complaints will be palpitation or breathlessness and apprehension.

This is the only wide-beat tachycardia you can treat with verapamil. It's perfectly safe in this specific form of tachycardia, and it usually stops the arrhythmia. In any other form of ventricular tachycardia, verapamil will probably cause ventricular flutter or fibrillation. Use of verapamil in any other type of ventricular tachycardia is malpractice. With this specific ECG configuration, it's perfectly safe and usually effective.

This peculiar tachycardia is probably *fascicular* — that is, it arises in the posterior fascicle of the left bundle branch, producing the typical right bundle–left axis configuration. It's caused by accelerated automatic discharge of an ectopic focus rather than by a reentry circuit, the

FIGURE 12-4

Mechanism of fascicular ectopic beats. (A) Beat arises in the posterior (left) fascicle of the left bundle at point A. It is conducted leftward along the posterior fascicle, causing an extreme left axis. (B) There is slow retrograde conduction into the right bundle. (C) As a result, some variety of right bundle-branch delay will be present.

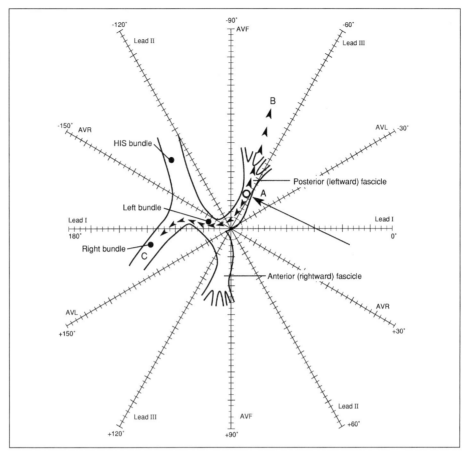

way most paroxysmal tachycardias are, hence the difference in prognosis and treatment.

Curious fact: When you administer verapamil for this type of tachycardia, the rate will slow progressively — e.g., 180–160–140–120–90–sinus. This is completely different from the all-or-nothing response of the common reentrant tachycardias and reflects the difference in the cause of the arrhythmia.

A combination of extreme right axis with right bundle-branch block almost certainly means an anterior fascicular tachycardia, but to date very few cases have been reported. Figure 12-7 is an example.

Note that when this kind of tachycardia arises in a patient with a compromised left ventricle, of course, it can be life-threatening simply because of the rapid, inefficient beating rather than because of the possibility of progression to a fatal arrhythmia.

Fascicular Beats and Fascicular Tachycardia **179**

I-II-III   aVR-aVL-aVF   V1-V2-V3   V4-V5-V6

FIGURE 12-5
Wide-beat tachycardia
with extreme left axis and
V1 configuration mimick-
ing right bundle-branch
block.

More recent electrophysiologic studies have proved that these tachycardias are indeed fascicular: When the right bundle–left axis pattern is
present, they originate in the posterior fascicle of the branch, exactly as
one would have predicted from the ECG configuration. Another related
type of ventricular tachycardia presents with a left bundle-branch pattern commonly with extreme inferior (rightward) axis deviation. This
has been shown to originate in the outflow tract of the right ventricle.

Both types of tachycardia are lumped under the title of "idiopathic
ventricular tachycardia" because they both appear in otherwise normal
hearts. In response to treatment, however, the two types of tachycardia
are radically different. As noted earlier, the right bundle–left axis variety
responds to verapamil, and it does so in a way that is unique: instead of
an abrupt ending of the tachycardia, there is stepwise reduction in rate
until the tachycardia disappears. The left bundle variety, however, responds to any of the usual drugs in the usual all-or-nothing manner.
Class I agents like lidocaine, quinidine, or procaine amide; beta blockers;
sotalol; and amiodarone are all moderately effective, and when treatment is successful the tachycardia stops at once.

FIGURE 12-6
Another wide-beat tachycardia with extreme left axis and a right bundle-branch block pattern in V1. In both these cases the patient's blood pressure remained normal and there was no serious hemodynamic compromise. Both responded to verapamil.

This and other data suggest that the two varieties of idiopathic ventricular tachycardia have a different mechanism. The right bundle–left axis variety is probably the result of enhanced automatic firing from a single focus, while the left bundle–right axis variety is probably the result of a small reentry circuit or "triggered" after depolarizations.

FIGURE 12-7
Wide-beat tachycardia
with right bundle-branch
block pattern and extreme
right axis. This is probably
a fascicular tachycardia
arising in the anterior fascicle of the left bundle, but
data on this configuration
are still sparse.

13 | Concealed Conduction, Exit Block, Bundle-Branch Wenckebach, and Supernormal Conduction

Concealed conduction and exit block are two conditions you can't actually see on the surface ECG; these are diagnoses you have to make in the great Sherlock Holmes manner by finding the only possible explanation for what's happening. They are definite entities, not flights of theoretical fancy; both abnormalities have been certified by electrophysiologic study and they're both important clinically.

Bundle-branch Wenckebach and supernormal conduction are both easy to recognize in the ECG, but they're very rare and often escape detection because physicians don't know they exist.

ECG Recognition of Concealed Conduction

Remember that conduction through the AV node is "silent" — that is, it doesn't produce any deflection on the surface ECG. Normally you measure conduction through the AV node by measuring the P-R interval, but sometimes the AV node is only partially penetrated. This can happen from above or below — that is, either sinus beats or ventricular ectopic beats can penetrate some distance into the AV node without going all the way through. How can you tell this has happened? Usually it's simple. The AV nodal tissues are unusually refractory when the next impulse comes along. This tells you they must have been partly penetrated and discharged.

The simplest example of concealed conduction into the AV node is what happens after a VPC. Often the VPC will penetrate the AV node without penetrating all the way through to the atria. The next sinus beat will find the tissues fatigued, and the first P-R after a VPC may be prolonged. Figure 13-1 is an excellent example.

FIGURE 13-1
Concealed conduction into the AV node from VPCs. The concealed conduction made the AV node refractory and produced the prolonged P-R. When the VPCs were eliminated, the P-R went back to normal.

FIGURE 13-2
Concealed conduction in the presence of a dissociated junctional rhythm. When the sinus impulse comes a sufficiently long time after the junctional beat, it finds the upper AV nodal tissue out of its refractory period. The sinus impulse penetrates to the site of the ectopic junctional pacemaker and resets it, hence the pause. The lower AV nodal tissues are refractory, so there's no conduction to the ventricles — just the pause in the junctional rhythm.

There are VPCs appearing every other beat, and the P-R of the sinus impulses is prolonged (0.29 seconds). When the VPCs were eradicated with lidocaine, the P-R interval became normal. Obviously the VPCs were sending an impulse up into the AV node that penetrated far enough into the nodal tissues to make them refractory when the next sinus impulse came along.

Figure 13-2 illustrates concealed conduction in the presence of a dissociated junctional rhythm. In the first part of the tracing, there is a junctional rhythm with dissociated P waves that come farther and farther after the QRS with each beat. After the third QRS there is an abrupt pause in the junctional rhythm, and then it resumes.

The ladder diagram shows what happened. The sinus impulse came *so long after the junctional beat* that it found the upper nodal tissues out of their refractory state and was able to penetrate the AV node far enough to reach the site of the junctional pacemaker and discharge it. That's why there's a pause in the junctional rhythm. This is *concealed conduction* with "reset" of a junctional pacemaker. None of the sinus impulses reach the ventricles because they arrive at the AV node when the cells below the site of the junctional pacemaker are still refractory.

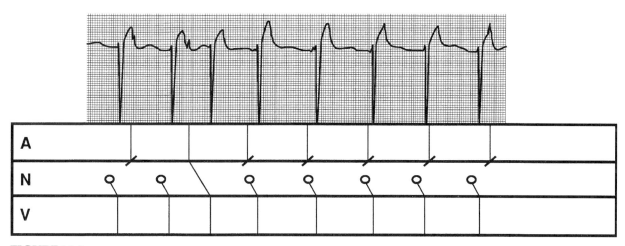

FIGURE 13-3
A dissociated junctional rhythm with one capture beat by the sinus node (the third beat on the strip).

FIGURE 13-4
Concealed penetration of the AV node by the sinus impulse. At "X" the sinus impulse penetrates to the site of the junctional pacemaker but doesn't penetrate the lower AV node to reach the ventricles. The evidence of the concealed conduction is the pause in the junctional rhythm.

Figures 13-3 and 13-4 provide another example of the same phenomenon. In Fig. 13-3 there is a dissociated junctional rhythm: After the second QRS the P wave comes late enough to find the AV nodal tissues ready to conduct and the sinus impulse "captures" the ventricles for one beat.

In Fig. 13-4 the same thing happens, except this time the sinus impulse doesn't get all the way to the ventricles. It does penetrate as far as the junctional pacemaker and resets it, causing the obvious pause. Thus you see concealed conduction into the AV node. You know it happened because there's a pause in the junctional rhythm, and the pause takes place every time the P wave comes a critical distance *after* the junctional beat so that the nodal tissues have recovered enough to permit penetration to the site of the ectopic pacemaker.

These last two examples of concealed conduction are important because they tell you that *the AV block in each case is not complete.* How do you know? Simple. The sinus node can penetrate to the site of the junctional pacemaker and reset it. The junctional pacemaker can obviously reach the ventricles, because it does so most of the time. Therefore, there is a potential functioning track from atria to ventricles. It's only a matter of timing.

Concealed conduction can also take place in the bundle-branch system, but this is usually not significant in clinical terms. On the other hand, concealed conduction in the AV node, as in the examples above, can be very significant indeed for the clinician trying to evaluate AV block.

Exit Block

You're familiar with block in the AV node and in the bundle-branch system. Now picture a kind of block in the tissue around the various pacemakers of the heart.

Start with the sinus node. The sinus node consists of two kinds of cells: the cells that form the activating impulse and those that conduct it out to the atria (Fig. 13-5). The activating impulse can encounter block in those conducting cells, just the way it can encounter block lower down, in the AV system. The difference is that this time you can't see the impulse in the activating cells; you can see it only when it reaches the atria and starts to form a P wave. This kind of block is called "exit block" because it keeps the impulse from making its exit into the conducting tissues. You can tell there's block because suddenly a P wave doesn't appear.

FIGURE 13-5
Diagram of pacemaker and conducting cells of the sinus node.

P	○ ○ ○ ○ ○ ○	The sinus node consists of pacemaking cells that generate an electric potential. (P cells)
C	↓↓↓↓	There are also conducting cells, that conduct the impulse out to the atria. (C)
A	When the impulse enters the atria, a P wave is produced.	

Failure of conduction in the "C" cells of the sinus node produces "exit block", preventing the sinus impulse from reaching the atria. This can take several forms.

FIGURE 13-6
Sinoatrial exit block with pauses that are precise multiples of the basic rate.

FIGURE 13-7
Exit block around the ectopic atrial pacemaker during PAT with block.

In the classic type of sinoatrial exit block, there's a sudden pause equal to exactly twice the basic rate, because the pacing cells of the sinus node go on firing normally. The problem is that one impulse doesn't reach the atria to form a P wave. The next impulse comes in right on time, so the pause equals a double interval, just like the pause in Mobitz-II block (Fig. 13-6).

Figure 13-7 illustrates typical exit block around the ectopic atrial pacemaker during PAT with block. Note that the pause is an exact double interval of the basic atrial rate. (This was the first case of its kind recorded: I was fortunate enough to run across it in our laboratory back in the early sixties.)

Figure 13-8 illustrates the Wenckebach type of exit block around the sinus node. This is a 3:2 ratio of conduction. Two pacing impulses reach the atria and produce P waves, but the third one is blocked. Therefore you see two P waves with pause. You know there's a Wenckebach type of exit block *because the pause is less than twice the basic rate.* Remember, that's typical of Type I block.

Accelerated idioventricular rhythms are common. So is exit block around the cells that cause the rhythm, down in the ventricular subendocardium. The block will most commonly be Wenckebach, or Type I. You'll remember that another characteristic of Type I AV nodal block is that as the P-R interval grows longer, the R-R interval, paradoxically, grows shorter. Of course that's because while the P-R grows longer, the

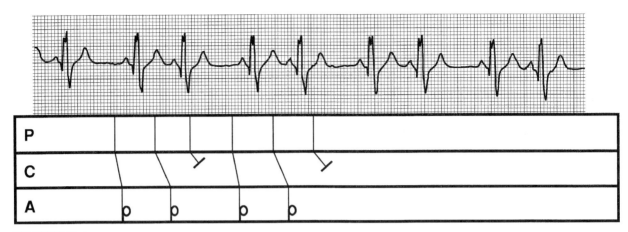

FIGURE 13-8
Sinoatrial exit block, Wenckebach type with 3:2 conduction to the atria.

FIGURE 13-9
Wenckebach type of exit block around an idioventricular focus interrupting atrial fibrillation. Note characteristic progressive shortening of R-R.

amount of increase is progressively smaller with each beat. P-R values might run 0.16–0.24–0.26–0.27 in a typical Wenckebach cycle. The same thing happens when there's Type I block in the tissues around an ectopic ventricular focus: You'll see a shortening R-R interval, typical of Type I block (Figs. 13-9 and 13-10).

When you see a pause, it may be less than double the R-R interval of the beats ahead of the pause, exactly like the pause after a blocked P wave in AV nodal Wenckebach (Fig. 13-10, top strip). In the bottom strip of Fig. 13-10 the progressive shortening of R-R in the four-beat runs of ventricular beats leaves no question that there's an exit Wenckebach block around the ectopic focus. (The pause here is longer than you'd expect with a typical AV nodal Wenckebach, but the time required for an ectopic focus to "recharge" and start firing again doesn't always fit a precise pattern.)

FIGURE 13-10
Variable periods of Wenckebach exit block around an idioventricular focus.

Bundle-Branch Wenckebach and Supernormal Conduction

Figure 13-11 illustrates two rare phenomena that can be confusing if you don't understand them. Here and there through the strip you see an obvious bundle-branch block. (It's lead I, so it has to be left bundle-branch block.) In the first beat on the left (1) you see intraventricular conduction delay but not a full-blown bundle-branch block. Beat 2 is left bundle-branch block, and beat 3 is a normal QRS! The interval between the left bundle-branch block beat and the normal beat is short. The normal beat in fact comes early, because it's a PAC. Next you have a VPC followed by two left bundle-branch block beats (4 and 5) and another PAC *with a normal QRS* (6). After this second PAC there's a pause and the next beat is normal (7).

Now you can begin drawing conclusions. First, beat 7 tells you that rate-dependent bundle-branch block is present, since the normal QRS appears after a pause. Next look at beats 8 and 9. Beat 8 is wider than 7, but it's not a full-blown bundle-branch block. In beat 9 you see complete bundle-branch block. In other words, *there's a progression from incomplete to complete left bundle-branch block.* Look at the last six beats on the middle strip and you see the same thing. There's progressive widening of the QRS until there's complete left bundle-branch block in the last three beats. These are Wenckebach periods within the left bundle. The impulse is conducted with progressive slowing, with more widening of the QRS until it isn't conducted at all: At that point, complete bundle-branch block appears. So far, so good: everything's reasonable. Now you see all the rules broken. Look at beats 3 and 6 in the top strip and beats 3, 6, and 9 in the middle strip. They're PACs. They come early — but the QRS is normal. The left bundle-branch block has disappeared! You can't explain

FIGURE 13-11
Combination of rate-
dependent left bundle-
branch block, Wenckebach
periods within the left
bundle branch, and super-
normal conduction in the
left bundle branch.

the narrow QRS on the basis of rate; the bundle-branch block appears at a rate of 90 and up, but the R-R interval ahead of the narrow beat is equivalent to a rate of 150. You can't explain the narrow beat on an Ashman basis because the R-R relation is exactly opposite to what you would expect. You can't invoke bradycardia-dependent aberrancy to explain the left bundle-branch block because the narrow beats, like beat 7 in the top strip, also come after a long pause. The only explanation for these narrow beats is the *supernormal phase of conduction.* This is a rare bird, but here it is. Just after the T wave there is sometimes a phase of supernormal conduction when you see conduction through tissues that are usually blocked — the left bundle in this case.

There's still no good electrophysiologic explanation, but the fact that it does occur is indisputable. Supernormal conduction probably occurs only in bundle-branch tissues. You will usually see it with rate-dependent bundle-branch block and bundle-branch Wenckebach periods, as in this example. In this setting you may see an early beat with normal conduction that you can't explain on any of the usual bases of intraventricular conduction. You have to invoke supernormal conduction. Although this phenomenon is described in all serious works on arrhythmias, it isn't even mentioned in the current major textbooks of cardiology. Pity.

Note to all residents and fellows: You hereby have my permission to copy this tracing and spring it on the attending at morning report. Do it with a casual air, saying something like "obvious, but interesting, don't you think?" (Theory and practice of roundsmanship!)

14 | Fatal Arrhythmias: Ventricular Fibrillation, Ventricular Flutter, Torsade, R-on-T Phenomenon, Standstill

Two arrhythmias can be instantly fatal: ventricular fibrillation and ventricular standstill. They're so simple to recognize that they hardly need any discussion.

Ventricular Fibrillation

When the ventricles fibrillate, the ECG records a disorganized set of deflections. These may be large or small, fine or coarse. Of course there aren't any P waves. These deflections are an accurate picture of what's going on in the heart muscle. When you look at a fibrillating heart or hold it in your hand, it's obvious that the muscle is quivering like a dying sea creature. There's absolutely no pumping activity of any kind (Figs. 14-1 and 14-2).

FIGURE 14-1
"Fine" ventricular fibrillation. The electric activity produces only minimal twitching in the baseline.

FIGURE 14-2
"Coarse" ventricular fibrillation. There is some evidence that coarse ventricular fibrillation, with large deflections like the ones illustrated here, is more likely to respond to cardioversion.

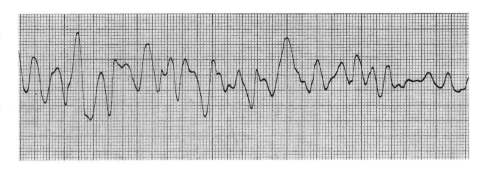

FIGURE 14-3
Ventricular flutter. Note the large, regular deflections with no distinction between QRS and T. This arrhythmia is equivalent to ventricular fibrillation: No blood is being pumped, and death is almost instantaneous.

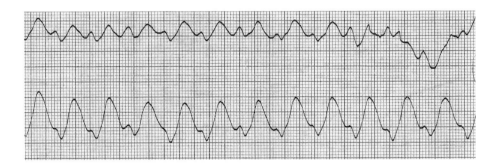

Ventricular Flutter

This is in fact a form of ventricular fibrillation that can be deceptive on the ECG. There are large, rapid, regular ventricular complexes that might make you think you were looking at ventricular tachycardia. The difference is that these complexes have no organized shape. You can't tell the QRS from the T because all you see is a simple wave: A physicist would call it a "sine wave." Ventricular flutter is the same as ventricular fibrillation in its effect on the heartbeat. The heart is twitching feebly but regularly. No blood is being pumped, and the victim dies almost at once unless the rhythm is changed (Figs. 14-3 and 14-4).

Torsade

We used to call this "polymorphic ventricular tachycardia," but then a French cardiologist coined the elegant name "torsade de pointes" because the changing of axis in successive beats made him think of a ballerina twisting on her toes — "sur les pointes." Glamorous foreign names have an unfair advantage, so that's the term we use now.

FIGURE 14-4
On the left-hand side of this strip there is well-defined ventricular tachycardia. On the right-hand side this degenerates into ventricular flutter, with large, formless regular waves.

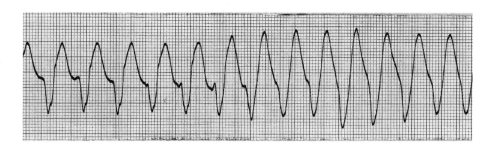

FIGURE 14-5
Torsade. The ventricular complexes are first upright, then isoelectric, then negative, and finally upright again as the axis of the ectopic beat "twists" around 180 degrees.

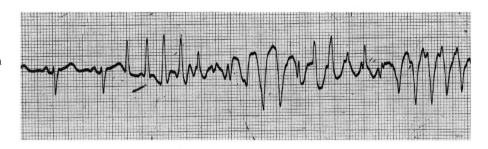

It's an important and dangerous arrhythmia. In torsade the shape of the QRS complexes changes rapidly and progressively from upright to isoelectric to negative and back to upright again. In fact the axis of the complexes really does "twist" around 180 degrees (Figs. 14-5 and 14-6).

It might be easy to mistake these for ventricular fibrillation, but you'll notice the progressive change in the QRS shape with reasonably well-defined QRS and T complexes. Torsade is usually brief, but if it's sustained it can be fatal. Torsade is often seen when the Q-T interval is prolonged; usually that's the result of drugs like quinidine. Rarely it's the result of a congenital abnormality of cardiac activation that produces lifelong prolongation of the Q-T interval. (If the prolonged Q-T is associated with congenital deafness, it's called the Lang-Jervil-Niellsen syndrome. If there's only Q-T prolongation, it's called the Romano-Ward syndrome.)

Treatment of torsade is completely different from treatment of ventricular flutter or fibrillation, and it's not covered in any of the usual texts or courses on cardiac resuscitation. Here it is:

1. Intravenous magnesium (2 g) are given by bolus, and a drip of 2 mg/min. is started at the same time.

FIGURE 14-6
Torsade. There are short bursts of torsade in both strips, with typical dramatic shift in axis of the ectopic beats. Note occasional abrupt prolongation of the Q-T in some beats just before a burst of torsade.

2. If torsade persists or recurs, accelerate the ventricular rate by atrial pacing. Drugs like atropine or isoproteronol would also work, but pacing's more reliable. Warning: Isoproteronol should never be administered when there's any question of myocardial ischemia: it's likely to lead to infarction or fatal arrhythmias. Atropine and pacing are simpler, safer ways of speeding the heart rate.

Between these two measures, torsade can be controlled 100% of the time.

Prevention: If the prolonged Q-T is caused by drugs, stop them. If it's congenital, treat with beta blockers.

If beta-blockers fail, resection of the stellate ganglion often succeeds. The congenital form of torsade seems to represent an imbalance of left and right sympathetic innervation so that resection of several left sympathetic ganglia has given very good results.

Finally, the perfection of implantable defibrillators has been a giant stride in the control of these arrhythmias. Defibrillators can be implanted with substantially no risk and with performance that is close to 100% in recognition and control of torsade. Torsade associated with congenital prolonged Q-T intervals may be the ideal indication for implantable defibrillators.

R-on-T Phenomenon

For many years everybody knew that sometimes an electric shock would put the heart into ventricular fibrillation, and sometimes it wouldn't. Why the difference? Bernard Lown and his associates answered the puzzle. There's one small fraction of time during the heart cycle when the heart is vulnerable: A shock delivered during that time will produce ventricular fibrillation. During the rest of the heart cycle the heart is relatively safe. This is the principle of elective cardioversion: The machine delivers the shock *outside* of the vulnerable zone. This vulnerable zone is about 0.01 seconds long and lies just ahead of the peak of the T wave (Fig. 14-7).

When a VPC hits the vulnerable zone of the T wave, it can act as an electric shock and cause ventricular fibrillation (Fig. 14-8). This is commonly described as the "R-on-T" phenomenon. We now know a good deal more about this phenomenon than we used to. The R-on-T phenomenon is important in only three specific settings:

1. In the presence of acute myocardial ischemia such as an infarct.
2. In the presence of a low serum potassium.
3. In the presence of a prolonged Q-T interval.

FIGURE 14-7
The vulnerable zone of the heart cycle is a tiny segment of time just before the peak of the T wave. It is about 0.01 seconds in duration.

FIGURE 14-8
Example of the R-on-T phenomenon triggering torsade. Note the VPC in the T wave of the last sinus beat before torsade begins.

In any other setting a VPC hitting the vulnerable zone isn't any more important than any other VPC.

Standstill

There's really nothing to recognize on the ECG. Anybody can tell that a flat line is flat. The manipulations going on during a cardiac arrest can produce many twitches in the baseline that might look like ventricular fibrillation. It's important to have everyone take their hands off the patient for a few seconds to see if standstill is in fact present. After all, the treatment for standstill is quite different from the treatment for ventricular fibrillation, so the distinction can be critical. Figure 14-9 illustrates a typical very slow idioventricular rhythm degenerating into standstill.

The treatment of ventricular fibrillation and ventricular standstill is so widespread in the various ACLS courses that there's no need to go into it here. (The surprising and somewhat shocking fact is that none of these courses teach how to treat torsade.)

Measurement of the Q-T Interval

The Q-T interval is important in fatal arrhythmias, specifically in torsade. It's time to learn how to measure it and to recognize abnormal prolongation.

The Q-T interval varies with the rate: the faster the rate, the shorter the Q-T interval, and vice versa. The Bazett formula was an attempt to establish a normal value corrected for rate. The expression "Q-Tc" means

FIGURE 14-9
Two idioventricular beats
ending in standstill.

"Q-T interval corrected for rate." Bazett attempted to correct for rate by the formula Q-T/square root of R-R. This gives an upper normal level of 0.39 seconds for men and 0.44 for women. The Bazett formula is relatively crude; Q-T intervals are best derived from the tables of Ashman and Hull, and Lepeshkin (Table 14-1).

Table 14-1 Normal variations of the Q-T interval

Heart Rate	Lower Limit	Upper Limit	
		Men & Children	Women
40	0.42	0.49	0.50
43	0.39	0.48	0.49
46	0.38	0.47	0.48
48	0.37	0.46	0.47
50	0.36	0.45	0.46
52	0.35	0.45	0.46
55	0.34	0.44	0.45
57	0.34	0.43	0.44
60	0.33	0.42	0.43
63	0.32	0.41	0.42
67	0.31	0.40	0.41
71	0.31	0.38	0.41
75	0.30	0.38	0.39
80	0.29	0.37	0.38
86	0.28	0.36	0.37
93	0.28	0.35	0.36
100	0.27	0.34	0.35
109	0.26	0.33	0.33
120	0.25	0.31	0.32
133	0.24	0.29	0.30
150	0.23	0.28	0.28
170	0.22	0.26	0.26

15 | The Sick Sinus Syndrome

The cells of the sinoatrial node are subject to all the slings and arrows of infection, ischemia, and degeneration. Disease of the sinoatrial tissues often produces an abnormally slow sinus rate. In extreme cases the sinoatrial node may "die," with total replacement of active cells by scar tissue.

When depression of sinus node function causes symptoms, the "sick sinus syndrome" is said to be present. Thus to diagnose the sick sinus syndrome, it isn't enough to read an electrocardiogram. You have to be a clinician: you have to take a history.

The diagnosis of sick sinus syndrome can be established only when abnormally slow discharge of the sinus node produces symptoms. If there are no symptoms, there is no syndrome, no matter how alarming the bradycardia may appear on the ECG.

At least 90% to 95% of the time, the symptoms of subnormal sinus node function will be *cerebral*. Inadequate perfusion of cerebral tissues may produce vertigo, "presyncope," or frank syncope. Less commonly, an inappropriately slow sinus rate may exacerbate or perpetuate congestive heart failure with symptoms ranging from generalized fatigue to incapacitating dyspnea. Very rarely, a sinus rate too slow to sustain circulation may cause ischemic pain — a kind of bradycardia-dependent angina. (I've seen only one case like this in the last thirty-plus years.)

ECG Diagnosis

Subnormal sinus node function can take one of three forms.

Inappropriate Sinus Bradycardia
This takes some careful defining. Normally, the sinus rate varies on demand within wide limits. Rates of 30 or 40 are common during sleep, while vigorous activity may produce rates of 150 or higher. "Inappropriate sinus bradycardia" means that the sinus rate is persistently too

low to support the circulation at any given level of activity. In other words, the sinus rate can be assessed only in terms of the immediate needs of the body. A rate of 40 or 50 might be adequate during sleep, but it won't support the circulation when the patient is climbing stairs.

Figure 15-1 illustrates severe, sustained bradycardia. The rate remained in the range of 40 even when the patient walked or performed other exercise that would normally increase the heart rate. With this persistently low rate the patient became dizzy and sometimes started to faint.

Sinus Pauses

The sinus node may suddenly pause so that there's no activity for several seconds or even longer. Sinus pauses are common; everybody has them. They are significant only if they produce symptoms.

(Cardiology, like the rest of medicine, is haunted by myths. The legend of the three-second pause ranks right up there with the tooth fairy for pure mendacity. An author of a text once made a casual comment that three-second pauses might be dangerous and might justify implantation of a pacemaker. This was no more than an offhand opinion, without supporting data. Large-scale studies subsequently proved that three-second pauses are common and harmless and should be disregarded unless they produce symptoms, but the genie was out of the bottle. Uninformed or unscrupulous physicians to this day persist in inserting unnecessary pacemakers on the basis of an occasional three-second pause even though the patient has no symptoms whatsoever.)

Sinus pauses can take one of two forms:

1. The first is true sinoatrial exit block. This is relatively rare. Suddenly there's no P wave and, of course, no QRS. The next beat comes in exactly on time. The pause is exactly double the basic rate — in other words, it's equal to two R-R intervals (Fig. 15-2). This precise double interval means that the pacemaking cells of the sinus node actually went on firing at regular intervals, but suddenly one impulse wasn't con-

FIGURE 15-1
Severe symptomatic sinus bradycardia recorded during light exercise (walking).

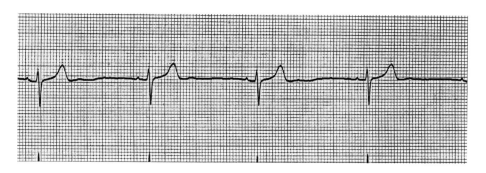

FIGURE 15-2
Sinoatrial block. The pauses are an exact multiple of the basic sinus rate. This means that the pacing cells of the sinus node have gone on building up their charge and discharging normally, but an occasional impulse isn't conducted out to the atria.

FIGURE 15-3
Random sinus pauses with no relation to the basic sinus rate.

ducted out to the atria. Go back to Fig. 13-5 and recall that there are pacemaking cells and conducting cells in the sinoatrial node. With this kind of block the pacing cells are normal, but the conducting cells occasionally fail.

2. Random sinus pauses are much more common. Suddenly there's no P wave and hence no heartbeat for a long time. The pause has no relation to the basic sinus rhythm (Fig. 15-3). Sometimes these pauses can come out of the blue, interrupting a normal sinus rhythm, and they can be very prolonged indeed.

If sinus pauses produce symptoms, and *if* they are recurrent and not drug-induced, a pacemaker will probably be needed.

FIGURE 15-4
Junctional escape beating. The slow sinus rate (40) permits the junction to escape and set the rhythm for several beats at a time. Note the occasional pairing, or "bigeminal," rhythm when a junctional beat is followed by a sinus beat. This is "escape-capture bigeminy," typical of sick sinus patterns.

FIGURE 15-5
AV nodal block associated with severe sinus bradycardia and occasional escape junctional beats. The AV block is actually first-degree, with P-R interval of 0.38 seconds. The occasional apparent short P-R is caused by junctional escape beats that have no connection to the preceding P waves.

Fortunately, the automatic-demand pacemakers in the junction and the ventricles are usually ready to pick up the rhythm if the sinus node fails. In Fig. 15-4 you see a sinus rate of about 40 with two junctional escape beats between successive sinus beats. When you see junctional or idioventricular escape beating, always check the sinus rate to see if an abnormally slow sinus rate is the reason for the "escape" of the ectopic focus.

In Fig. 15-5 there is evidence of AV nodal block together with long sinus pauses and junctional escape beating. AV nodal block commonly accompanies sick sinus behavior and may be a reflection of the same pathologic process. All the hallmarks of the sick sinus are present in this tracing: Now you have to ask the patient about symptoms!

The Bradycardia-Tachycardia Syndrome
Sometimes periods of slow sinus rhythm are interrupted by bursts of abnormal rapid rhythms in the atria — flutter, fibrillation, or atrial tachycardia. It's common to have a patient present with one of these tachyarrhythmias and then convert to an abnormally slow sinus rate or to one interrupted by frequent long pauses (Figs. 15-6 and 15-7).

The Sick Sinus Syndrome **201**

FIGURE 15-6
Bradycardia-tachycardia syndrome. A run of PAT is followed by severe, symptomatic sinus bradycardia.

FIGURE 15-7
Bradycardia-tachycardia syndrome with atrial flutter as the "tachy" component. Note the sustained bradycardia when the sinus rhythm resumes.

FIGURE 15-8
Not the brady-tachy syndrome. There are paroxysms of coarse atrial fibrillation with a perfectly normal sinus rhythm and rate between paroxysms. This patient can safely be treated with suppressive drugs like quinidine or procaine amide. No pacemaker needed.

FIGURE 15-9
Pseudoblock. Severe sinus bradycardia, rate 40, with "escape" of a junctional pacemaker. Note occasional sinus capture beats, such as the beat produced by the second P wave in the bottom strip. Two capture beats are also apparent in the top strip. These capture beats tell you that this is interference-dissociation caused by the slow sinus rate — it is *not* complete AV block.

This is the bradycardia-tachycardia form of the sick sinus syndrome. What causes this combination of events? It is possible that the absence of sinus node impulses for long periods allows the abnormal rapid rhythm to "take over," although this cannot be the entire explanation.

Caution: To diagnose the bradycardia-tachycardia syndrome, you have to document significant periods of bradycardia between the episodes of tachyarrhythmia. Don't diagnose a "brady-tachy" syndrome just because you see paroxysms of flutter, fibrillation, or tachycardia. In most cases you'll see periods of normal sinus function between episodes of tachyarrhythmia. Be sure you document symptomatic bradycardia before you diagnose the brady-tachy syndrome.

Figure 15-8 illustrates this point. Here you see paroxysms of atrial fibrillation with short periods of sinus rhythm. This is *not* a brady-tachy phenomenon because there's no "brady." There are three sinus beats in V1 and two in V2; these sinus beats appear at a rate of about 80 to 88, indicating normal sinus node function.

A variant of brady-tachy is "pseudoblock" with the sick sinus syndrome. In Fig. 15-9 there's a severe sinus bradycardia, rate about 43. This slow rate permits a junctional pacemaker to "escape," setting the rhythm of the heart until a sinus beat arrives between ectopic beats and captures the rhythm of the heart momentarily.

Important: Even though there are periods of complete AV dissociation, there's no AV block — just a dearth of P waves. This particular patient didn't need a pacemaker; he just needed relief from the toxic drugs

The Sick Sinus Syndrome   **203**

that were suppressing his sinus node (clonidine and digitalis in this case).

The Mystery of the Sick Sinus Syndrome

Normally the "demand" ectopic pacemakers in the junction and in the ventricles will set the rhythm if the sinus node fails. In the sick sinus syndrome, they often don't. That's why there are long pauses and that's why symptoms appear. If the subsidiary pacemakers functioned normally, there would be no symptoms, hence no syndrome. In the sick sinus syndrome there is really a failure of all pacing systems from the sinus node to the ventricles; nobody has even come close to explaining how or why this happens.

Caution: It's safe to say that more than 90% of all cases of subnormal sinus node function are caused by physicians. There's an alarmingly long list of drugs that can depress sinus node function:

Digitalis
Quinidine
Procaine amide
Calcium blockers
Beta blockers
Clonidine
Morphine and other opium derivatives
Psychotropic drugs
All the newer antiarrhythmic drugs, such as amiodarone, sotalol, and propafenone

The sinus node may be temporarily depressed during myocardial infarction. Retching and vomiting can stimulate the vagus with some spectacularly long pauses. Hyperkalemia typically slows the sinus node; so does hypothyroidism. In other words, be sure to rule out the effect of drugs or other metabolic abnormalities before you decide the sinus node itself is "sick." True sick sinus syndrome is rare. In our busy county hospital, where many of our patients are old and sick, I might see only one genuine sick sinus syndrome in a year.

The sick sinus syndrome isn't usually a threat to life. One large-scale British study was unable to find a single case of cardiac arrest caused by the sick sinus syndrome. There are anecdotes of rare cases of cardiac arrest caused by sinus node failure, but there is no authenticated list of such occurrences in the world medical literature. (Obviously the sick sinus syndrome is a threat to life if it causes syncope while someone is driving a car!)

The only treatment of the sick sinus syndrome is permanent pacing. When the brady-tachy syndrome is present, it's also essential to treat the tachyarrhythmia with suppressive drugs.

Occasional happy outcome: When a patient has paroxysms of atrial fibrillation as part of a brady-tachy syndrome, the physician should pray that the atrial fibrillation becomes permanent. When that happens, the sinus node is irrelevant and the treatment is the same as for any ordinary case of atrial fibrillation. No pacemaker is needed, since there are plenty of fibrillary impulses bombarding the AV node. All the physician has to do is to control the rate.

The diagnosis of the sick sinus syndrome is made by recording an ECG during symptoms. This can be done by an ordinary ECG, by an event recorder, or by Holter recordings. The event recorder has been a boon: It can be worn for two weeks, can record up to fifteen episodes, and has a five-minute memory loop. In other words, it is now *always* possible to record an ECG during symptoms. An ECG recorded during symptoms is the gold standard — no other studies are necessary.

In past years there were attempts to measure sinus node function by invasive means, but these were never very sensitive and are now totally obsolete. If some invasive EP enthusiast wants to study your sick sinus syndrome, bar the door and burn his catheter. Invasive EP studies have no place in the modern diagnosis of the sick sinus syndrome.

16 | Digitalis-Toxic Arrhythmias

In recent years the uses of digitalis have become precisely defined. Digitalis can slow the ventricular rate by depressing AV nodal conduction, it can suppress atrial and junctional ectopic activity, and it is a mild inotrope. Digitalis may also be the most overused drug in the world. It's often prescribed in a kind of knee-jerk clinical reflex for old sick people who don't really need it, and it often does more harm than good. Specifically, it causes arrhythmias, some of them dangerous; in the current jargon, it is powerfully proarrhythmic. Digitalis-toxic arrhythmias are much less common than they were a few years ago, but they still emerge with distressing frequency. They're dangerous!

Figure 16-1 explains the double-toxic effect of digitalis. First, it stimulates the vagus nerve. Second, it "turns on" ectopic firing anywhere in the heart. Remember, the vagus nerve is the "slowing" nerve in the heart. When the vagus nerve is overstimulated, it can depress the sinus node so that it fires very slowly and sometimes stops firing entirely. In other words, digitalis can produce a sick sinus syndrome (Chap. 15).

Diagnosis of Digitalis Toxicity: The Four Commandments

Commandment One

If you see subnormal sinus node function in a patient taking digitalis, *always* assume that digitalis toxicity is the cause.

Overstimulation of the vagus nerve can also produce block in the AV node. This is a very common effect of digitalis toxicity. AV block caused by digitalis is always localized in the AV node, never in the bundle-branch system. The reason for this is simple: Digitalis produces block in the AV node by stimulating the vagus nerve. The vagus nerve doesn't reach the bundle-branch system. It stops around the bottom of the AV node (Fig. 16-2).

FIGURE 16-1
The double-toxic effect of
digitalis.

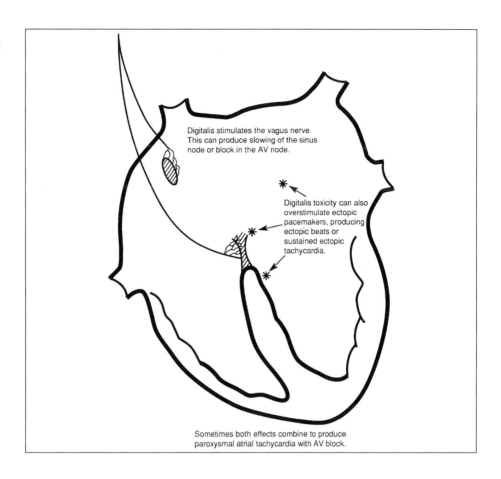

Digitalis stimulates the vagus nerve.
This can produce slowing of the sinus
node or block in the AV node.

Digitalis toxicity can also
overstimulate ectopic
pacemakers, producing
ectopic beats or
sustained ectopic
tachycardia.

Sometimes both effects combine to produce
paroxysmal atrial tachycardia with AV block.

FIGURE 16-2
Vagus nerve anatomy. The
fibers of the vagus nerve
reach the AV node and may
penetrate the bundle of
His. Vagal fibers do not
reach the bundle-branch
system. Block produced by
vagal stimulation will
therefore always be localized in the AV node.

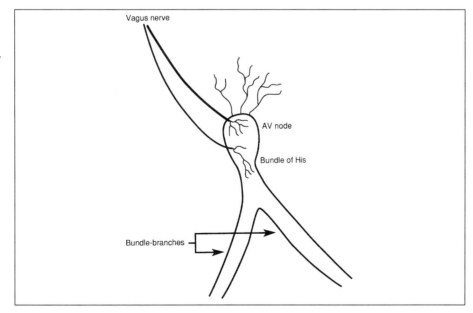

Vagus nerve

AV node

Bundle of His

Bundle-branches

Digitalis-Toxic Arrhythmias **207**

Digitalis toxicity can produce any type of AV nodal block — first-degree, 2:1 or other "fixed ratio," Type I (Wenckebach), and complete block.

You will *never* see Mobitz-II block as a result of digitalis toxicity, because Mobitz-II block never occurs in the AV node. Since the vagus nerve does not send fibers to the bundle-branch system, digitalis toxicity has no effect on the bundle-branch tissues, where Mobitz-II block takes place.

Commandment Two

When you see AV nodal block in a patient on digitalis, *always* assume that digitalis toxicity is the cause.

Digitalis-toxic AV nodal block is always temporary. The immediate antidote is atropine. Sometimes temporary pacemakers are necessary.

The other effect of digitalis toxicity is a kind of stimulation of ectopic foci anywhere in the heart — atria, junction, or ventricles. Ectopic firing as single beats or as sustained tachycardia will be the result.

The VPC is the most common single arrhythmia caused by digitalis toxicity. When frequent VPCs appear in a digitalized patient, especially if they start forming couplets or triplets, it's a good bet that digitalis is the cause. It's also a good time to stop the digitalis to see if the beats go away.

Commandment Three

Any ectopic beats that appear in a digitalized patient should be assumed to be the result of digitalis effect. This is especially important if the ectopic beats are ventricular.

Commandment Four

This is a golden rule. You'll save lives if you learn it and observe it: Certain types of paroxysmal tachycardia in a digitalized patient should always be regarded as digitalis-toxic until you prove otherwise. On the other hand, some types are never the result of digitalis toxicity.

For instance, AV nodal reentrant tachycardia will never be the result of digitalis toxicity, nor will AV nodal reciprocating tachycardia (bypass tract) or true ectopic atrial tachycardia of childhood.

On the other hand, whenever you see accelerated junctional rhythms, ventricular tachycardia, or paroxysmal atrial tachycardia with AV block in a digitalized patient, the diagnosis is digitalis toxicity until you prove otherwise.

1. Rapid junctional rhythms are the most common type of digitalis-toxic sustained tachycardias. These rhythms may appear in several forms. Figure 16-3A illustrates a true paroxysmal junctional tachycardia with a rate of 148. Figure 16-3B illustrates an accelerated junctional

FIGURE 16-3

(A) Paroxysmal junctional tachycardia, rate 150. (B) Accelerated idiojunctional rhythm, rate 90. Both are examples of digitalis-toxic junctional rhythms.

V1-V2-V3 V4-V5-V6

A

B

rhythm with a rate of 90. Both rhythms were the result of digitalis toxicity. Thus digitalis toxicity may produce either an accelerated junctional rhythm in the high-normal range or a true paroxysmal junctional tachycardia.

2. Ventricular tachycardia is of course the most dangerous type of digitalis-toxic paroxysmal tachycardia. It looks exactly like any other kind of ventricular tachycardia; you make the diagnosis by taking a history.

Digitalis Levels

AV nodal block or paroxysmal tachycardia caused by digitalis can be diagnosed only by discovering that the patient is taking digitalis and making the assumptions listed above. Digitalis levels in the blood are useful only to tell you that the patient has in fact been taking the drug.

Serum levels of digitalis (digoxin) do not correlate with toxicity or with therapeutic effect. The patient can be toxic at low levels (0.9

ng/mL) or subtherapeutic at high levels (2.8–3.0 ng/mL). You make the diagnosis of digitalis toxicity from the history and the ECG findings.

One more time: In everything described so far, you make a clinical assumption. If AV nodal block or certain types of paroxysmal tachycardia appear in a patient taking digitalis, you assume that digitalis is the cause until it's proved otherwise. Why is all this so important? The digitalis-toxic tachyarrhythmias are very dangerous. As an overall risk, it's conservative to say that giving more digitalis will produce a 36% mortality.

PAT with Block

Now we come to a dangerous digitalis-toxic arrhythmia that you can recognize from the ECG. It's a combination of the two elements in Fig. 16-1, that is, acceleration of an atrial ectopic focus together with AV nodal block.

Look at Fig. 16-4. You see P waves coming rapidly and regularly with a rate of 214. Every other P wave is blocked. There is 2:1 AV nodal block. (You know the block is in the AV node because the QRS is narrow.) These are the two elements in this critical diagnosis: PAT with block. Remember, to make the diagnosis you note first that P waves are appearing rapidly and regularly. Therefore there is a paroxysmal atrial tachycardia. Now you make another simple observation: Not all the P waves are reaching the ventricles. Therefore there is some degree of AV block. That's all you need to know. The block may be first- or second-degree, of any of the usual nodal types. The type of block isn't important.

Remember the two simple elements in the diagnosis of PAT with block:

1. You see rapid, regular P waves in the tachycardia range.
2. Some of the P waves are blocked.

PAT with block is caused by a combination of digitalis toxicity and a low serum potassium about 90% of the time. The treatment is intravenous potassium, administered rapidly. More digitalis at this point is likely to be fatal.

FIGURE 16-4
Paroxysmal atrial tachy-
cardia with 2:1 AV block.

Figures 16-5 through 16-9 illustrate variations of PAT with block. Notice that the ventricular rate can be fast or slow, regular or irregular, depending on the atrial rate and the degree of block. It could be very easy to confuse this with atrial fibrillation.

FIGURE 16-5
PAT with block. In the first five beats the P-R prolongs progressively until one P wave is blocked. The sixth beat is a junctional escape beat, and then a three-beat Wenckebach cycle follows. Wenckebach periods are present through the rest of the tracing. Note the irregular ventricular response as the degree of block changes.

FIGURE 16-6
PAT with variable block. On the right-hand side of the strip you'd have a hard time making a diagnosis. On the left side you can see P waves very clearly; the atrial rate is 210. There's obviously atrial tachycardia. Not all the P waves reach the ventricles, so there is AV block. That's all you need for the diagnosis of PAT with block. If you march the rest of the P waves out you can see that there are P waves hidden in the QRS complexes on the right-hand side of the strip with a variable degree of AV block. The exact type of block isn't important; what *is* important is that there is atrial tachycardia with some kind of AV block.

FIGURE 16-7
PAT with block. The degree of block is variable, ranging from 3:1 to 6:1 in various parts of the strip. The two essentials for the diagnosis are obvious: (1) there are P waves appearing rapidly and regularly in the paroxysmal-tachycardia range, and (2) they don't all reach the ventricles. That's all you need to see to diagnose this very dangerous arrhythmia.

FIGURE 16-8
This illustrates a number of types of AV block with PAT. In the top strip there are periods of 2:1 block that shift into Wenckebach cycles with a 3:2 response. The bottom strip begins with a 4:3 Wenckebach period and shifts to first-degree block with a P-R of 0.30 seconds. It's hard to see the P waves buried in the P waves during 2:1 block, but the changing shape of the T waves during Wenckebach periods makes it clear that there's a P wave hidden in them. This gives you the clue to the atrial rate — about 128.

One of the silliest medical myths is that an "irregular irregularity" of the heart means atrial fibrillation. By now the student should be able to list a half-dozen other arrhythmias that can cause "irregular irregularity" of the heart beat. PAT with block is one of them.

If you decided that the rapid irregular rhythm in Fig. 16-4 was caused by atrial fibrillation and gave more digoxin, the patient would probably die. Any intelligent jury would call it malpractice. You'd have no defense.

Special distinction: The thoughtful student will note that there are similarities between atrial flutter and PAT with block. In each there's a rapid abnormal regular atrial rhythm. In each there's some kind of failure of conduction to the ventricles. Thus, it might be easy to confuse them.

However, there are several important differences. The diagnosis of flutter is made by detecting typical flutter waves in the ECG. The atrial

FIGURE 16-9
PAT with 2:1 block interrupted by PVCs. Warning: Except for the PVCs, this is a slow regular rhythm with a rate of 80. It would be impossible to distinguish this from a normal sinus rhythm at the bedside! Rely on the ECG and always be suspicious when patients are on digitalis.

waves of PAT are typical separate P waves with an isoelectric period between them. The atrial flutter rate can be very fast. If you see an atrial rate of 300 in the adult, it has to be flutter. PAT never goes that fast; in fact, PAT very rarely goes over 250. Flutter is almost never a digitalis-toxic arrhythmia. PAT with block almost always is. Digitalis is an excellent treatment for flutter; it's lethal with PAT with block.

Study Fig. 16-10 carefully because you will certainly have to make the distinction between these two arrhythmias. The wrong answer can be fatal.

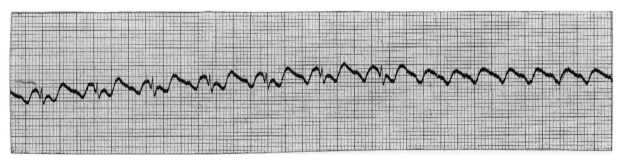

FIGURE 16-10
Typical flutter waves. At the right-hand end carotid sinus pressure has been applied to block conduction through the AV node; the flutter waves are seen without QRS complexes. Note how the end of one wave is the beginning of the next. There is no flat, or isoelectric, period between waves. Compare these typical flutter waves with the P waves in Figs. 16-3 through 16-8. Even though the atrial rate is in the same range as the flutter rate, there is no mistaking the well-defined P waves with a flat, or isoelectric, period between them.

Digitalis Toxicity and Atrial Fibrillation: A Very Special Case

Practically every case of atrial fibrillation is treated with digitalis, and it's safe to say that most cases of digitalis toxicity appear in exactly this setting. It's extremely important, therefore, to be able to recognize digitalis toxicity in the presence of atrial fibrillation. If you remember what digitalis does, it's not difficult.

Digitalis-Induced AV Block in the Presence of Atrial Fibrillation

In incomplete block, there will be no P waves to measure from, so you simply go by the rate. Figure 16-11 is an example of atrial fibrillation with a very slow ventricular rate. The rhythm is irregular, so you know that the fibrillating impulses are still driving the ventricles, but they're coming through the AV node so slowly that common sense tells you there's a high degree of block. Stop the digitalis!

The diagnosis of complete AV block in the presence of atrial fibrillation is simple (Fig. 16-12). The ventricular rhythm is regular, and the rate is 45 or less. The regular ventricular rhythm tells you that there's com-

FIGURE 16-11
Atrial fibrillation with high degree of AV nodal block and frequent VPCs.

FIGURE 16-12
Atrial fibrillation with complete AV nodal block and VPCs forming a "bigeminal" rhythm.

plete AV dissociation — in other words, an "idio" pacemaker is driving the heart, and none of the fibrillating impulses are coming through the AV node. The slow rate tells you that the block is complete. (Another one of those beautiful, high-fidelity golden oldies from my intern days!)

Interference-Dissociation and AV Block

Remember the phenomenon of interference-dissociation back in Chap. 7. You'll often see the same thing when the atria are fibrillating and there's incomplete block in the AV node. Conduction from the atria slows just enough to let an ectopic focus in the AV junction or in the ventricles "escape" and set the rhythm of the heart. In Fig. 16-13 you see atrial fibrillation. The first beat, marked "f," is conducted from the fibrillating atria; so are the other beats marked "f" later in the tracing. Most of the time you see a regular rhythm with wide QRS complexes ("V"). This is an idioventricular rhythm. It tells you that there's some degree of block in the AV node, but the occasional conducted beats tell you that the block is not complete.

When the pulse turns regular in a fibrillating patient, look out! It doesn't necessarily mean that you've restored a sinus rhythm. If the pulse is slow and regular, there's probably complete AV block. If it's regular in the normal range, there may be an idiorhythm with partial AV block. In either case the patient is digitalis-toxic.

FIGURE 16-13
Atrial fibrillation interrupted by long runs of an idioventricular rhythm (V), rate 60. A few beats are conducted from the fibrillating atria (f). There is a high degree of block, not complete.

Ectopic Beats

Ventricular ectopic beats are the most common single manifestation of digitalis toxicity in the ECG. Figure 16-14 is typical. When VPCs begin appearing frequently or in couplets, assume digitalis toxicity.

Paroxysmal Tachycardia

When the rhythm turns regular and the rate is rapid, paroxysmal tachycardia is interrupting the atrial fibrillation. You recognize junctional and ventricular tachycardia just the way you do in any other setting (Figs. 16-15 and 16-16).

FIGURE 16-14
Atrial fibrillation interrupted by many multifocal VPCs, ending in ventricular fibrillation. This is a graphic illustration of the possible fatal outcome of digitalis toxicity.

FIGURE 16-15
Digitalis-toxic ventricular tachycardia interrupting chronic atrial fibrillation.

FIGURE 16-16
Digitalis-toxic long runs of junctional tachycardia interrupting chronic atrial fibrillation. Note the regularity of the complexes and occasional periods of aberrant conduction. The tachycardia appears in runs of varying length, so the pulse has periods of irregularity. Bedside distinction from atrial fibrillation would be very difficult.

Diagnostic Algorithm for Digitalis Toxicity in the Presence of Atrial Fibrillation

Here's an "algorithm" or systematic approach to detecting digitalis toxic rhythms in the fibrillating patient.

A. Rhythm irregular, rate slow. Incomplete AV block.
B. Rhythm regular, rate slow to normal, three possibilities:
   1. Normal sinus rhythm has been restored.
   2. Atrial fibrillation persists with complete AV dissociation. Check an ECG at this point!
      a. If rate is 45 or less: complete AV block.
      b. If rate is in the normal range, an idiorhythm is present with partial AV block.
C. Rhythm regular, rate rapid (140 or more): paroxysmal tachycardia is present.

Unless a normal sinus rhythm has been restored, all the other possibilities listed above mean digitalis toxicity!

Tips on Treatment

There's no specific drug therapy for digitalis-toxic supraventricular tachycardia. Make sure electrolytes, especially K and Mg, are in the high-normal range, and support the patient until the digitalis wears off. If the tachycardia threatens life, treat with specific antibodies, such as FAB fragments. Remember, you can do this only once in the patient's lifetime, so be sure it's needed! I've never had to use it.

The specific therapy for digitalis-toxic ventricular tachycardia is *intravenous diphenylhydantoin*. The effect is specific, immediate, and gratifying. This is the only arrhythmia that responds to diphenylhydantoin. One good protocol is 100 mg slow push q five minutes until the arrhythmia ends *or* toxic CNS symptoms appear *or* a gram has been given. Then go to maintenance.

Potassium for PAT with block should be given relatively rapidly — 10 meq per hour or even more if the patient is severely distressed.

17

Myocardial Infarction

It's sound practice to start with pathophysiology. Myocardial infarction, of course, is always caused by abrupt occlusion of a coronary artery. In most cases this is the result of thrombus formation in a diseased vessel. Rarely, an atheroma can be "levered out" by subintimal bleeding so that it blocks the artery totally even without a thrombus. Even more rarely a thrombus can form in an apparently normal artery. Spasm in an anatomically normal artery can cause total occlusion with infarct formation, and with distressing frequency, the combination of spasm and accelerated atheroma formation in cocaine addicts can kill young people in their 20s and 30s. For whatever reason, the artery is occluded, and within seconds, electrophysiologic changes take place in the insulted myocardial cells.

You may remember crushing a frog's gastrocnemius in the physiology laboratory and recording an "injury current." That's exactly the same kind of current that's generated in acutely ischemic myocardial cells (Fig. 17-1). If you were to place an electrode on the epicardium directly over the injured area, you'd record an S-T deviation: The S-T segment would be elevated (Fig. 17-2). The injury current registers during the S-T segment because the balancing currents introduced by the electrocardiogram offset the injury current during the rest of the heart cycle.

Now comes an extremely important principle in ECG diagnosis of myocardial infarction: If you were to go around to the other wall of the heart, exactly 180 degrees from the site of the occlusion, you'd record depression of the S-T segment (Fig. 17-3). This illustrates the phenomenon of image cancellation. In plain language, whatever you record on one side of the electric field of the heart can be recorded upside down on the opposite side. It's like a mirror image, except that it's not right to left — it's upside-down. Changes seen on the side of the heart opposite the site of the infarct are called the *reciprocal* pattern. Changes recorded directly over the infarct site are called the *infarct* pattern.

FIGURE 17-1
A thrombus occludes a
diseased coronary artery.
The changes of ischemia
begin within seconds.

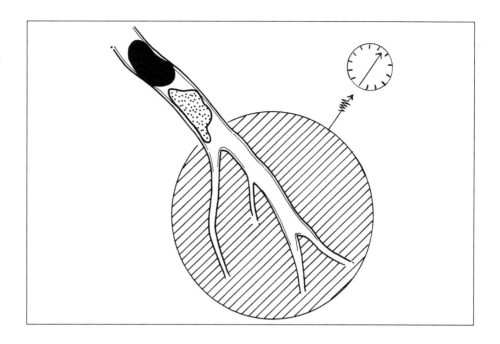

FIGURE 17-2
The acutely ischemic tis-
sue produces an injury
current — a small, steady
potential that registers
during the S-T segment. In
the lead that "faces" the
infarct, the S-T segment
will be elevated.

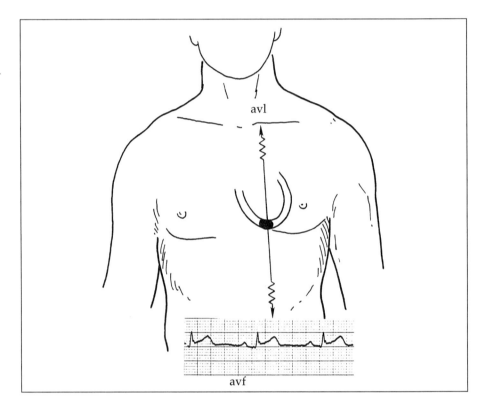

Stay with the lead "facing" the infarct for the time being. Suppose it's an inferior infarct and you're looking at avf. If you stood at the junction of the thigh with the trunk and looked straight up you'd be looking at the inferior or diaphragmatic surface of the heart, and that's exactly what avf records (Fig. 17-4). The S-T elevation may be a millimeter or less or it may be very high indeed — 5–10 mm or more (Fig. 17-5).

FIGURE 17-5
Varieties of S-T elevation with myocardial infarction.

FIGURE 17-6
Further progression of S-T change with upward "coving" of the S-T segment and beginning inversion of the T wave.

In Fig. 17-6 there's a further progressive change. You'll note that the S-T segment has an upward concavity. This curve is called the "Pardee cove-plane curve" after the man who described it. Our interns describe this as the "tombstone" curve, and it's not a bad term, all things considered.

Distortion of depolarization may be the next change. As the cells undergo the changes of ischemia, there is dispersion and slow conduction of the depolarizing impulse. This will of course distort the depolarizing impulse with change in the QRS. The most common and most specific form of QRS distortion is the initial negative deflection or Q wave. In Fig. 17-7 the central shaded area represents the zone of early necrosis where the Q wave probably originates. When you see a combination of a pathologic Q wave with S-T elevation and beginning T wave inversion, you have an absolutely specific ECG diagnosis of myocardial infarction. A "pathologic" Q wave is one that is 0.04 seconds wide. Many older studies emphasized the depth of the Q wave compared with the R in the same lead, but careful pathologic correlation has proved that it is

FIGURE 17-7
The pathologic Q wave presumably arises from distortion of electric forces in the necrotic "core" of the infarct.

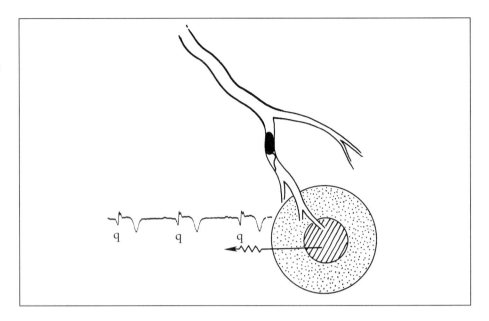

FIGURE 17-8
Varieties of pathologic Q waves. The important point is that they're both 0.04 seconds wide. Note beginning inversion of T waves.

the *width* of the Q that is important. Look at Fig. 17-8. The Q in the bottom strip is much deeper than the one in the top strip, but both are wide — at least 0.04 seconds wide — and that's what makes them pathologic Q waves.

Sooner or later all the injured tissue either dies or recovers. Either way, the injury current disappears and the S-T segment returns to the baseline. As this happens, the T waves progressively change shape in a direction opposite to the S-T deviation. This "opposite deviation" is what distinguishes the S-T-T pattern of infarction from that of hypertrophy.

FIGURE 17-9

"Stable" stage of evolution of an infarct pattern with Q, S-T segment almost back to baseline, and inverted T waves.

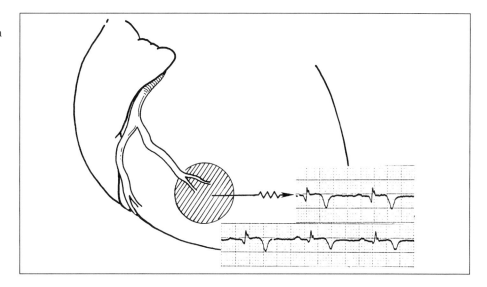

FIGURE 17-10

A simple way to visualize reciprocal patterns: The ECG recorded from one side of the electric field of the heart (A) will be seen in an upside-down mirror image on the other (B).

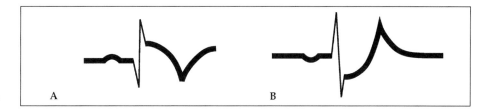

Figure 17-9 represents the "stable" stage of evolution of a myocardial infarct. The S-T segment was elevated, but now it's back to baseline and the T wave is inverted. This whole process may take minutes, hours, or days. The whole evolution may be complete in 24 hours or it may take as long as two weeks. This last fact is important to note. Studies by Gorlin and others have shown that the evolution of the ECG in an ordinary, uncomplicated myocardial infarct may take as long as two weeks. Don't become anxious and start thinking of catheters just because there's still some S-T deviation after a week or so. This is well within the range of normal.

You're now ready to apply the principle of reciprocal deviation or "upside-down image" to the diagnosis of myocardial infarction. Just to make sure you're clear about what the reciprocal pattern is, try drawing the full-blown ECG of myocardial infarction, complete with Q wave, elevated S-T segment, and inverted T wave (Fig. 17-10). Now turn the paper back to front and upside down and look at it against the light. Where "A" is you see the pattern inscribed in "B" and vice versa. In "B" you

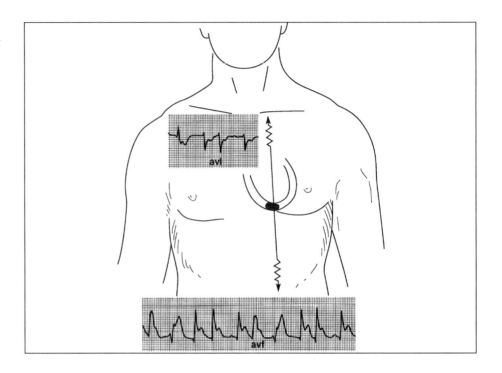

recognize that instead of a Q wave you see an R; instead of an elevated S-T segment you see one that's depressed; instead of an inverted T wave you see one that's upright. This is the reciprocal pattern of infarction and it's just as important as the "direct" infarct pattern in diagnosis. From here on we're going to use the terms *infarct pattern* and *reciprocal pattern:* Be sure you understand what they mean.

Now look at Fig. 17-11. There is very striking S-T elevation in avf, leaving no doubt that there's acute ischemia in the inferior wall. Note the reciprocal pattern in avl, exactly opposite the deviation in avf. You diagnose an inferior myocardial infarct, therefore, when you see infarct changes in the "left leg" leads — II, III, and avf. You confirm the diagnosis when you see reciprocal changes in the leads that are 180 degrees opposite — I and avl.

When you see reciprocal changes like these, the diagnosis of acute myocardial infarction is established with 100% confidence. (It's unfortunate that the investigators in the various studies of thrombolysis in myocardial infarction didn't include anybody with a primary interest in electrocardiography. They produced criteria for thrombolysis like "2 mm S-T elevation in adjacent leads" but totally overlooked the most specific S-T-T deformity for infarction — the reciprocal deviation described here. Most experienced electrocardiographers will agree that the finding of reciprocal S-T-T changes together with significant symptoms is much more specific than simple S-T elevation.)

A Critical Point About Q Waves

A pathologic Q wave is one that's 0.04 seconds wide. Q waves this wide are always abnormal and practically always indicate necrotic change in the myocardium, new or old. Go back to Chapter 5 and look at Fig. 5-1 to refresh your memory about normal, physiologic septal Q waves. Remember that activation of the septum normally produces a narrow Q. The rules are simple:

1. A Q wave that's 0.02 seconds wide is normal, or "septal."
2. A Q wave that's 0.04 seconds wide is pathologic.
3. A Q wave that's 0.03 seconds wide is borderline, possibly pathologic.

Keep a hand lens handy, because you're going to be measuring hundredths of a second.

With These Basic Elements You're Ready to Detect an Infarct and Localize It Anatomically

Here are the basic rules.

Anterior Infarcts
The infarct pattern is present in the precordial leads. There are usually no reciprocal changes because you can't record from the opposite, or posterior, aspect of the left ventricle (Fig. 17-12). Anterior infarcts can be usefully divided into anteroseptal (V1 and 2, possibly 3) and anterolateral (V5 and 6). (See examples later in the chapter.)

1. Inferior infarcts: Infarct pattern in II, III, and avf; reciprocal pattern in I, avl (Fig. 17-11).
2. Lateral infarcts: Infarct changes in I, avl, sometimes in V5, 6; reciprocal pattern in II, III, avf (Fig. 17-13).

Posterior Infarcts
These can be diagnosed only by finding the reciprocal pattern in the precordial leads, since the posterior wall of the heart can't be recorded directly by the ECG (Fig. 17-14). Note the tall R in V1 — it's really an "upside-down" Q. The depressed S-T segments are the reciprocal recording of elevated S-T segments on the other side of the electric field of the heart. Often inferior infarcts will include the posterior wall: When

FIGURE 17-12
Anterior MI. Q waves, elevated S-T segments, and inverted T waves in V1–4.

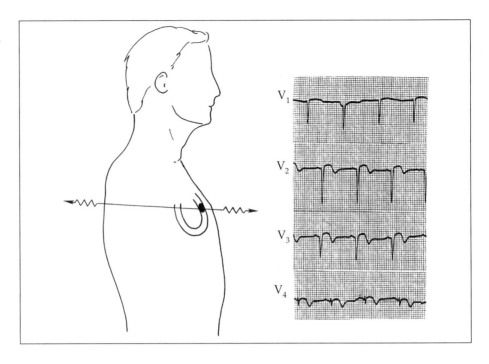

FIGURE 17-13
"High" lateral MI. Infarct pattern in avl, reciprocal pattern in avf.

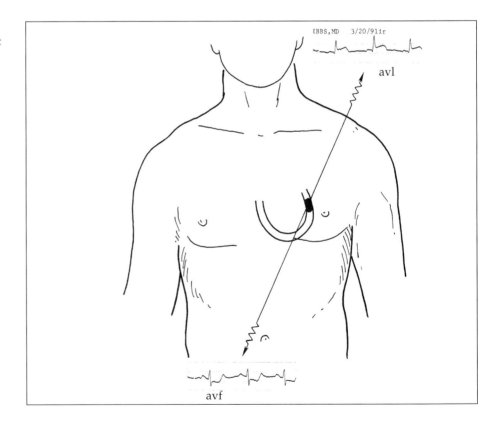

FIGURE 17-14
Posterior-wall MI. You
can't record directly over
the posterior wall, so you
have to rely on the reciprocal pattern in the right precordial leads—V1–3.

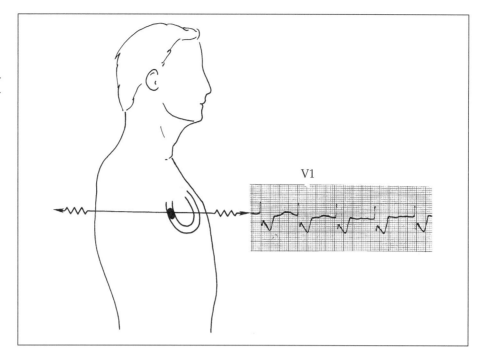

there are infarct changes in II, III, and avf with reciprocal changes in V1, 2, or 3, there is an inferior-posterior combination (Fig. 17-15). This is an important combination of findings to recognize because it usually means there's a great deal more jeopardized myocardium than in a simple inferior MI. Later in the chapter you'll have a chance to study a series of examples of infarction, illustrating a number of variations from the basic infarct patterns described above.

At this point a little recent medical history must be cleared up. With all this talk about "reciprocal changes," some of you may be thinking back to studies published ten or more years ago suggesting that these "upside-down" S-T relations were really the result of remote, coincidental ischemic events in a different coronary artery. Some investigators looked at coronary angiograms recorded at the time of infarction, and of course, they found disease in other coronary arteries as well. That's not surprising: It's safe to say that in about half of all infarcts there is multiple vessel disease. These investigators concluded that reciprocal changes were the result of two coincidental ischemic processes evolving at exactly the same time, with identical but opposite S-T changes hour by hour and even minute by minute. If you think about that very long, you're confronting a staggering coincidence. Subsequent investigations have established the "reciprocal" basis for S-T deviation and cleared the air of the "remote-coincidental" phenomenon; in fact, in the last edition of

FIGURE 17-15
Infarction of inferior and
posterior myocardium.
This is a common combi-
nation.

Braunwald, Fisch rejects the notion entirely, but there may still be echoes
around to worry the student. Forget it.

Special note on right ventricular infarction. Infarction of the right ventricle will always occur in association with the ECG pattern of inferior
myocardial infarction. In addition, right precordial leads can be diagnostic. These are recorded from positions over the right precordium that
are analogous to the left-sided leads. Thus, V4-R is recorded in the right
mid-clavicular line and so on. The ECG diagnosis of right ventricular infarction in these leads is simple: Any S-T elevation of 1 mm or more in
the right precordial leads is both sensitive and specific for right ventricular infarction. The typical "cove-plane" or "tombstone" configuration
will appear, just as in the left-sided leads.

Some Commandments About the ECG and the Diagnosis of Myocardial Infarction

1. Don't overread! The ECG may help you diagnose an infarct but it won't tell you how large it is or how dangerous it is, or whether it's subendocardial or transmural. A patient can go into cardiogenic shock with one inverted T wave, whereas another patient with S-T elevation all across the precordium may hardly be aware that anything's happened. You can't prognosticate from the ECG!

2. You've been looking at typical examples of infarction. Remember that you may see only fragments or parts of these patterns — one deviated S-T segment, one deformed T wave, one pathologic Q. If the symptoms are typical or even suspicious, any acute change in the ECG should be regarded as supporting evidence in the diagnosis of myocardial infarction.

3. Don't forget the distinction between normal septal Q waves and pathologic Q waves.

4. One more time: The evolution of an MI may be complete in a few hours or it may take two weeks. Don't overreact if the ECG evolves slowly; unless there are symptoms or other signs of further ischemic insult there's no reason to intervene. (In this day of the overanxious catheter, that's a very important bit of advice.)

5. When are wide Q waves normal? In two places: V1 and sometimes V2 and in lead III.

The right precordial leads "look down" into the negatively charged cavity of the heart, and many normally record a QS — much the same as the potential recorded in avr. On the other hand if V1 has a small R wave, and if the leads to the left — such as V2, 3, or 4 — *then* record a Q, that Q is 100% diagnostic of infarction.

Since the earliest days of electrocardiography, it has been known that Q waves and inverted T waves are found in lead III in about 15% of normal individuals. It wasn't until Goldberger invented the unipolar limb leads that we understood why that happened. Avl and avf actually record the electric potential at the left shoulder and the left thigh. Lead III is based on the difference between those two points. When the left leg — avf — is positive compared to the left arm — avl — there's an upstroke in III. When avf is negative compared to avl, lead III records a downstroke. "Negative" also can mean simply "less positive."

Suppose you have a 2-mm R in avf and an 8-mm R in avl. Avf is less positive than avl, so there's a downstroke, or Q, in III. This is a "false" Q based on the fact that avl is recording a higher potential than avf. This problem doesn't arise in I and II because the indifferent electrode is avr,

FIGURE 17-16
Q wave equivalent. The tall R in V1 is in fact an "upside-down" Q.

FIGURE 17-17
Q wave equivalent. A new tall R appears in avl and a new deep S in avf, reflecting loss of inferior forces in an inferior-wall MI. The axis has shifted superiorly, away from the infarcted area.

which is all negative. For practical purposes, ignore lead III and look at avf. That's the actual left leg potential and that's all you need to see.

Q Wave Equivalents

A Q wave is a deformity of the initial forces of depolarization that emerges as a negative deflection in the surface ECG. Will this deformity always appear as a negative deflection? Of course not. It can appear as a positive deflection, depending on the lead being recorded — such as the tall R in V1–2 in posterior infarction. In fact, myocardial infarction can distort any part of the QRS and it can do it in many different ways.

When you think of the varieties of location and type of pathology associated with myocardial infarction, it's obvious that a whole spectrum of changes can be produced in the QRS. The middle and terminal forces of the QRS can be distorted just as easily as the initial forces. The surface ECG can show gain or loss of potential, difference in speed of inscription, and change of direction. Many investigators have recorded these changes, and they can be lumped under the heading of "Q wave equivalents." If you're not prepared to recognize them you'll miss critical diagnostic information. The notion that infarction will distort only the initial forces of the QRS and that it will always produce a negative deflection has been described as "electrocardiographic naivete," yet many studies comparing "Q wave" and "non-Q wave" infarcts have been based on this crude distinction.

Types of Q Wave Equivalent Deformities

1. The tall R in the right precordium with posterior infarction is the best-known and most widely accepted Q wave equivalent (Fig. 17-16).

2. A drastic shift in frontal-plane axis is another common change with infarction. Typically, an inferior infarct produces a loss of inferiorly directed forces so that the R in avf becomes smaller and the R in avl becomes taller, with a leftward and superior shift of axis toward the remaining viable myocardium (Fig. 17-17).

3. Striking localized loss of R in the precordial leads is widely recognized as a Q wave equivalent (Fig. 17-18).

4. Notching or slurring of various elements of the QRS is common (Figs. 17-19 and 17-20).

FIGURE 17-18
Q wave equivalent.
Abrupt loss of precordial R
voltage in the presence of
an anterior infarct.

FIGURE 17-19
Q wave equivalent. Loss of
R in avf in one day during
the course of an inferior
myocardial infarct, reflecting loss of viable inferior
myocardium.

232 Myocardial Infarction

FIGURE 17-20
Q wave equivalent. The previous day, avf had consisted of a tall R and avl of a small r followed by a deep S. Twenty-four hours after inferior infarction, avf is a tiny, slurred complex and avl has changed to a simple tall R.

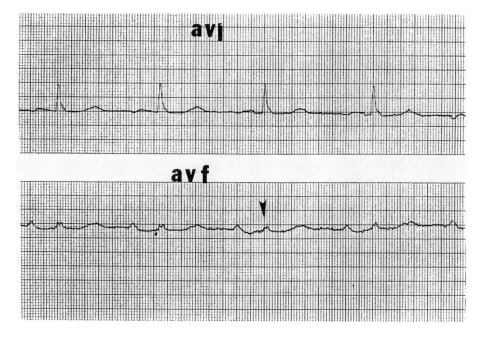

5. Sudden, otherwise unaccountable shift of axis — to the right in this case. This can be produced by a lateral-wall MI as a simple result of loss of leftward-conducting myocardium (Fig. 17-21).

Death of a Myth

You may have heard that Q wave infarcts are transmural and non-Q wave infarcts are subendocardial. There was never any basis for this notion; it was based on a mistake by Prinzmetal, which he later acknowledged. Every careful pathologic study has shown that about half of all Q wave infarcts are in fact subendocardial and about half of all non-Q wave infarcts are transmural. The Q wave tells you there's an infarct but it doesn't tell you anything about the pathology. I had the pleasure of helping to lay this myth to rest in one of the first editions of the *Journal of the American College of Cardiology* back in 1983.

(Special final note: When is avl significant and when isn't it? As you know, avr normally records a totally negative complex because it's recording a "cavity" potential. Sometimes avl records the same kind of potential because of a "vertical" heart (Fig. 17-22). When avl looks like avr, you can ignore the negative deflections. On the other hand, when avl is recording from left of the septum, you'll see the usual septal Q followed by an R or a plain tall R. A pathologic Q wave appearing in that setting of course is a very specific marker of infarction.)

FIGURE 17-21
Q wave equivalent. The ECG had been normal two weeks previously. Now the axis has shifted dramatically to the right, and there's a striking loss of R in V5 and V6 together with a tall R in V1. All these QRS changes are as significant as the presence of a simple pathologic Q: They mean infarction.

The last part of the chapter, from Fig. 17-23 to Fig. 17-41, presents a variety of ECGs recorded in the course of documented myocardial infarcts. These tracings illustrate a number of the possible variations and combinations of the simple elements presented so far. Take time to review them carefully.

FIGURE 17-22
"Cavity" potential in avl. Avl looks exactly like avr, which means that the avl electrode is recording from the negatively charged interior aspect of the left ventricle. The configuration of the QRS in avl therefore has no practical significance in this setting.

FIGURE 17-23
Note Q waves in V2–4.
The whole QRS complex
consists of a simple downward deflection, or Q
wave. This is sometimes
referred to as a "QS" complex. There is S-T eleva-
tion in V2–5 and
beginning T wave inver-
sion in V2–5 together with
an inverted T avl. Diagnosis: anterior myocardial infarction with lateral-wall
involvement (avl).

FIGURE 17-24

Q waves in II, III, avf, and V6. Elevated S-T segments in the same leads as well as in V5. S-T depression, avl. This is a typical pattern of inferior myocardial infarction with the infarct pattern in II, III, and avf and the reciprocal pattern in avl. It is very common for the infarct pattern to appear in V5–6 in inferior infarcts because the artery supplying the inferior myocardium almost always supplies the lower lateral wall of the left ventricle. It's important to realize that the changes in II, III, and avf and V5–6 are all part of the same process, *not* parts of two separate infarcts.

FIGURE 17-25
Typical reciprocal S-T deviation with elevation in II, III, avf and depression in I and avl. Seeing these leads alone you can predict inferior infarction with 100% accuracy.

FIGURE 17-26
V leads for tracing shown in Fig. 17-25. There are tall R waves in the right precordium with deeply depressed S-T segments, indicating infarction of the posterior wall with equal accuracy. (Turn these leads upside-down in your mind's eye and you see what you'd record if you applied an electrode directly to the posterior wall over the infarcted area.)

FIGURE 17-27
Q waves, I, avl, V2–5. Elevated S-T avl, V2–5. Evidence of anterior and lateral MI. Important point about Q waves: There's a small r in V1. This r disappears in V2–5, and true Q waves appear. Sometimes there's a QS complex in V1 or V2 simply because of the electric "position" of the heart, but when you see an rS complex in the right precordial leads, such as in V1, and then the r disappears and Q waves appear in the leads to the left of that point, it's 100% evidence that these are pathologic Q waves and that you're dealing with an anterior myocardial infarction.

FIGURE 17-28
Deep Q waves ("QS complexes") in V1–3. Elevated S-T segments V1–3. Beginning inversion of T waves in the same leads. Typical deformity of an anteroseptal MI.

FIGURE 17-29
Q waves and elevated S-T segments in I and avl. Reciprocal pattern in II, III, and avf. This is a true "high lateral" infarct in sharp contrast to the "low lateral" deformity in V5–6 often seen as part of inferior infarction.

FIGURE 17-30
"Hyperacute" S-T-T changes. (How can something be more acute than acute? Bad semantics but a useful term.) Dramatic S-T elevation in V2–3 with tall, upright T waves. This is a reliable indicator of acute anterior MI.

FIGURE 17-31

Now put together some of the things you've learned. There's a regular ventricular rhythm, rate 41. The QRS complexes are narrow. The P waves have no relation to the QRS complexes. Diagnosis: (1) complete AV dissociation with junctional rhythm, (2) ventricular rate less than 45, and (3) no capture by an adequate number of P waves to test the system. Conclusion: Complete heart block in the AV node (narrow QRS). Depressed S-T in I, avl; elevated S-T in II, III, avf; Q in III, avf. Inferior MI. (AV nodal block is common with inferior MIs because the artery that supplies the inferior surface also supplies the AV node about 85% of the time.)

FIGURE 17-32
Tiny r in V1. QS in V2–3. Inverted T in V1–4. Anteroseptal MI — almost always an LAD lesion.

FIGURE 17-33
Here's an infarct pattern developing before your eyes in about 23 seconds. This is lead V4, recorded during chest pain. Note the change in shape of the T wave from upright to inverted and back to upright across the top strip. Across the bottom strip you can see the typical injury current emerging with "tombstone" S-T elevation progressing to T wave inversion within five heartbeats. It can happen fast!

Myocardial Infarction   **245**

FIGURE 17-34
Another example of extreme S-T elevation in the early stage of an infarct. The top strip suggests bundle-branch block, but as you can see in the bottom two strips, there's simply extreme S-T elevation, so high that the S-T segment takes off from the top of the R wave.

FIGURE 17-35
"Hyperacute" S-T elevation in V2–4; reciprocal S-T depression in II, III, and avf.

FIGURE 17-36
High lateral MI with infarct changes confined to I and avl. Interesting configuration of avr with tall R: This is a reciprocal manifestation of the Q avl.

FIGURE 17-37
Precordial leads with a variation of the hyperacute pattern. Q waves are present from V1 through V5. Note interesting beginning of reciprocal S-T-T change in V6.

FIGURE 17-38
This is an extreme example
of hyperacute S-T-T deformity. Note also absence of
P waves with an acceler-
ated junctional rhythm interrupted by PVCs.
(Oddly, this patient subsequently had an uneventful
course; the initial appearance of the ECG can be really deceptive in terms of
the subsequent course.)

FIGURE 17-39
Q waves and Q wave equivalents everywhere — QS complexes from V1 through V5 plus avl (Q wave equivalent low voltages in frontal-place leads). This is one time you can do some prognosticating: really widespread Q waves connote a large area of infarction.

FIGURE 17-40
Minimal but dangerous! S-T depression in the precordial leads of the resting ECG raises four possibilities: digitalis effect, low serum K, hypertrophy, or ischemia. When you've ruled out the first three, *always* assume that precordial S-T depression means ischemia. This is a point not sufficiently emphasized by many authors, but it's absolutely reliable.

FIGURE 17-41

Here's the same phenomenon of precordial S-T depression, much more pronounced than in Fig. 17-40. It is further reinforced by reciprocal S-T in V6. It's important to remember that you can see reciprocal S-T deviation in opposite precordial leads, such as V1 and V6. This is sometimes a really important marker for infarction.

18 | Diagnosing Myocardial Infarction in the Presence of Bundle-Branch Block

Myocardial Infarction in the Presence of Right Bundle-Branch Block (RBBB)

This is easy. Most infarcts take place in the left ventricle. Since the left ventricle is activated normally whcn RBBB is present, you read the ECG the way you always would — with two obvious differences. First, you ignore the terminal wide deflection that characterizes RBBB — the wide terminal R in V1 and the wide terminal S in I and V6. Those wide deflections are, of course, the result of the conduction defect and have nothing to do with infarction. Second, remember that it's normal to see inverted T waves over the blocked ventricle. In other words, you expect to see inverted T waves in the lead with the wide terminal R — usually V1 and V2 and occasionally V3. Again, this T wave inversion is a result of the conduction defect and is a normal part of RBBB (Fig. 18-1).

Otherwise, you use exactly the same criteria for infarction you'd use if the RBBB weren't present. A Q wave is still a Q wave and has exactly the same significance with or without RBBB. You read the changes in the S-T-T complex exactly the way you always would. As you can see in Figs. 18-2 and 18-3, there are obvious pathologic Q waves, and the characteristic "tombstone" S-T-T deformity is obvious even in leads over the blocked ventricle.

Important Note about T Waves and RBBB
Although it's normal to see inverted T waves over the blocked ventricle, you should not see inverted T waves when you start recording over the left ventricular area — that is, when you're recording from V4, 5, or 6. When you lose the wide terminal R wave, you've left the electric field of the blocked ventricle. T waves to the left of this point should be upright. If the T waves are inverted over the normally activated ventricle, it's abnormal (Fig. 18-4).

FIGURE 18-1
Normal T wave configuration in RBBB. Note that the T waves are inverted only in the precordial leads with the wide R' — in other words, over the blocked ventricle.

FIGURE 18-2
Anterior myocardial infarction in the presence of RBBB. Note pathologic Q waves in II, III, and avf as well as in V1–6. The characteristic "tombstone" S-T elevation with reciprocal T wave inversion is present across the precordium. In other words, all the ECG elements of myocardial infarction are obvious despite the RBBB.

Sinus tachycardia; Rate 125, PR 14, QRS 12, right bundle branch block
Q V1,2,3,4,5,6, there is evidence of a new or extended anterior MI, that
was an extension of the previous process which now envolves an entire anterior
myocardium. This is a very bad prognostic sign together with right bundle branch
block.
BRENDAN PHIBBS, MD 6/4/91im

Rhythm[II] 10mm/mV

FIGURE 18-3
Striking changes of anterior myocardial infarction in the presence of RBBB and atrial fibrillation, with Q waves in V2–5 and unmistakable "tombstone" S-T-T pattern in the same leads.

FIGURE 18-4
Abnormal S-T-T configuration in the *left* precordial leads in the presence of RBBB. The T wave deformity in V1 and V2 can be attributed to the conduction defect, but from V3 to V6 the electrodes are clearly recording from the unblocked, or left, ventricular aspect of the field and the T waves should be upright. If they're not, the ECG is abnormal (arrows) and is consistent with myocardial pathology on some basis.

Myocardial Infarction in the Presence of Left Bundle-Branch Block (LBBB)

This is much more difficult and sometimes impossible to diagnose. Much of the time all you can say is that left bundle-branch block is indeed present, and that's the end of it (Fig. 18-5). However, there are sometimes clues that are very precise:

1. Any pathologic Q wave is still a significant Q even in the presence of LBBB (Figs. 18-6 and 18-7). LBBB per se never produces a pathologic Q; when you see one it's *always* the result of pathology and never the result of the conduction defect.

2. There's a specific kind of S-T-T deformity that characterizes LBBB. The S-T-T forces are directed away from the QRS forces so that in the lead with the wide R wave, there's a depressed S-T segment and a diphasic or inverted T (Fig. 18-8). However, you may see patterns of S-T-T deformity that don't fit the LBBB configuration. Sometimes you'll see a typical "tombstone" S-T-T in the presence of LBBB and then you can diagnose an acute ischemic process despite the presence of LBBB (Fig. 18-9). In other words, there's a kind of S-T elevation or depression you expect to find as a result of the LBBB. When you encounter S-T elevation or depression that doesn't fit the pattern of LBBB you can diagnose ischemia. Therefore, in the leads with a wide R wave like I, avl, and V6 you should see S-T *depression* as a result of the bundle-branch block. When you see *elevation* in these leads, it's never the result of the conduction defect; it indicates ischemia. Conversely, in leads with wide S waves like V1, 2, and 3, LBBB should produce S-T *elevation*. When you see S-T *depression* in these leads it's a very reliable marker of acute ischemia.

With all this in mind, take a look at Fig. 18-10 and you'll recognize a typical infarct pattern in III and avf, complete with pathologic Q waves and typical "tombstone" S-T-T. You can now diagnose myocardial infarction with perfect confidence despite the LBBB.

Figures 18-11 and 18-12 are striking examples of obvious myocardial infarction in the setting of RBBB and LBBB, respectively. As this book

I-II-III   aVR-aVL-aVF   V1-V2-V3   V4-V5-V6

Rhythm [II] 10mm/mV

FIGURE 18-5
Typical LBBB. The S-T-T
deformity is obviously
consistent with the con-
duction defect.

was going to press, a study of over 21,000 cases of myocardial infarction confirmed these observations about diagnosing LBBB in the presence of myocardial infarction, especially with reference to S-T depression in leads V1–3 in the setting of LBBB; the conduction defect itself never produces S-T depression in those leads.

FIGURE 18-6
LBBB with pathologic Q
waves in II, III, avf, and
V5–6. These are in fact
"QS" complexes. Note par-
ticularly that in V1–4 there
are R waves. When these
disappear with the change
to a QS complex in V5 and
V6, there is hard-core,
100% evidence of infarc-
tion or comparable pathology. The QS deformity
cannot possibly be attributed to the conduction
defect.

I II

III AVR

AVL AVF

A

FIGURE 18-7A and B
Pathologic Q waves in
leads I, avl, and V6 in the
setting of LBBB. This is
100% reliable as a marker
of lateral-wall MI. Note
also the typical "tomb-
stone" deformity of S-T
V6.

B

FIGURE 18-8
LBBB with very striking S-T-T deformity of the type consistent with the conduction defect. Note again the depressed S-T and inverted T "hockey-stick" configuration in the leads with the wide R, and the opposite configuration in the leads with the wide S. Contrast this with the "tombstone" S-T-T in the preceding illustrations; the difference is striking and diagnostic.

FIGURE 18-9
Comparison of the S-T-T pattern of LBBB with the "tombstone" S-T-T superimposed on preexisting LBBB (arrows). When the typical S-T-T pattern of infarction appears in the presence of LBBB, it is possible to make a precise diagnosis despite the conduction defect.

FIGURE 18-10
Obvious pattern of inferior
myocardial infarction in
the setting of LBBB.

FIGURE 18-11
Acute anterior ischemic S-T changes in the setting of RBBB. The S-T elevation V2–5 is totally different from the pattern you'd expect with RBBB. Note also the reciprocal S-T deviation in II, III, avf, and avl.

FIGURE 18-12
Striking hyperacute S-T-T deformity of anterior myocardial infarction in the presence of LBBB. Note also reciprocal S-T deviation with elevation in I and avl and depression in II, III, and avf.

19 | Transient Myocardial Ischemia and Angina Pectoris

Angina pectoris is a *symptom;* to be more precise, it's a collection of symptoms. Transient myocardial ischemia, on the other hand, is a *pathologic state.* It means that there's a temporary lack of adequate blood flow to some area of heart muscle. Sometimes transient myocardial ischemia produces the kind of discomfort we call angina pectoris. Sometimes it doesn't.

What are the symptoms of transient myocardial ischemia? To quote Ernest Hemingway, they're various. In the first place, there may not be any symptoms at all. Transient myocardial ischemia may be totally "silent." TMI (as we may now call it) may depress left ventricular function acutely, causing any or all of the symptoms of left heart failure. TMI may cause arrhythmias and can lead to sudden death. In other words, TMI can produce a whole spectrum of different signs and symptoms; classic angina pectoris is only one (Table 19-1).

The ECG is useful in transient myocardial ischemia in two ways:

1. It may demonstrate change during anginal symptoms, thus confirming the clinical diagnosis of angina pectoris.

2. It may demonstrate change when there are no symptoms, or when the symptoms are atypical, thus providing objective evidence that coronary artery disease is in fact present.

Table 19-1 Symptoms of transient myocardial ischemia

1. Angina pectoris
2. Transient depression of LV function with typical symptoms of congestive heart failure
3. Arrhythmias
4. "Nonspecific" symptoms — e.g., apprehension, paresthesias
5. Sudden death
6. Nothing ("silent" ischemia)

Transient myocardial ischemia is exactly what the name implies: transient. So are the ECG changes that accompany it.

The common ECG change during TMI is S-T deviation — elevation or depression (Figs. 19-1A, B, and C). There may also be deformity of the T waves — they may change from upright to inverted, or vice versa (Fig. 19-2). (The reader may recognize this as the first part of Fig. 17-33, recording the S-T-T changes in the seconds immediately before an MI.)

There are no specific S-T-T changes that characterize TMI; any acute change can be significant. The point to remember is that TMI sometimes produces change in the S-T-T complex and even in the configuration of the QRS. The absence of acute change doesn't rule out angina, but the presence of ECG change during pain is the strongest possible evidence of an acute ischemic process.

So far so good, but now the reader comes up against an odd gap in modern cardiologic knowledge: What is the specificity and sensitivity of acute S-T-T change in detecting TMI? Nobody can really answer this question because nobody's ever done an adequate study of the subject. When a patient lying in a hospital bed suffers pain that may be anginal, the nearest nurse will always administer nitroglycerine long before there's time to record a 12-lead ECG. That's as it should be: You'd have to be pretty cold-blooded to stand around watching a patient suffer

FIGURE 19-1
Examples of S-T deviation during transient myocardial ischemia, in these cases manifested by anginal pain. The S-T elevation is obvious in A. The minor S-T elevation in B is equally significant because it represented a change, during symptoms, from the baseline S-T previously recorded. On the left side of C there is typical "horizontal" S-T depression of 4 mm, diagnostic of ischemia. The upsloping S-T depression on the left side is less significant, but when changes of this magnitude accompany symptoms, the diagnosis of transient myocardial ischemia is established, for all practical purposes.

FIGURE 19-2
Very dramatic changes in
both S-T and T wave mor-
phology taking place
within a few seconds dur-
ing anginal pain. These
strips are continuous.

while you waited for the ECG machine to be connected just to let you
carry out some research! This small practical point has precluded any
definitive study of S-T-T change during spontaneous angina. Everybody
assumes that acute ECG change during pain is highly specific for TMI,
but how sensitive is it? How often does the ECG remain normal during
genuine spontaneous angina? Nobody knows.

In contrast to the ignorance that surrounds the question of S-T change
during spontaneous angina, there is voluminous information about the
kind and degree of S-T change during deliberate stress — e.g., during
stress testing. Certain reliable, well-correlated rules have emerged:

1. Any S-T elevation caused by physical stress is significant. It practically always connotes ischemia.

2. S-T depression is usefully divided into two types: "junction" depression and "horizontal or downsloping" depression.

3. Junction depression means that only the junction of the S-T with
the QRS is depressed; the rest of the segment slopes *upward* to the T
wave (Fig. 19-3). Junction S-T depression during exercise is significant
only if the depression is very severe — that is, if it equals 4 mm or more.
It's also necessary to take into account the *rate of rise* of the S-T segment.
If it's still depressed 2 mm or more, 0.08 seconds from the QRS, it's significant. In either case, this type of marked junction depression usually
connotes ischemia (Fig. 19-4).

FIGURE 19-3

FIGURE 19-4
Deep junction S-T depression. When the junction of the QRS with the S-T segment is depressed 4 mm or more, it has a high correlation with ischemia.

4. "Horizontal or downsloping" depression means that the S-T segment is depressed with a horizontal or downsloping configuration for at least 0.08 seconds from the junction (Fig. 19-5). When this kind of depression is present, the following numbers apply:

 a. 0.5 mm depression: possibly ischemia (odds about 50%).

 b. 1 mm depression: probably ischemia (odds about 75%).

 c. 1.5 mm to 2 mm depression: almost certainly ischemia (odds about 90%).

These criteria have been assessed against angiographically demonstrated coronary artery disease in many thousands of cases, so there's no question that they're reasonably reliable in the right setting.

So far so good, and all very scientific, but what about S-T-T changes appearing during spontaneous angina? Do the same criteria apply? What about S-T changes in the absence of symptoms? What exactly do they mean? Nobody knows. There are really no good studies on the subject and indeed it's a very difficult subject to study if you think about it for a moment. Here are a couple of reasonable rules. *Any* acute S-T elevation during anginal discomfort should be considered evidence of ischemia. The same is probably true of any acute S-T depression appearing during pain: As far as anybody knows, this is true whether the depression is junctional or horizontal-downsloping. The distinction used in stress testing probably doesn't apply here. Roughly speaking, the more pronounced the deviation from baseline, the more reliable the diagnosis of ischemia.

What about T wave changes? This is really a mystery. Everybody is sure that T wave change may be evidence of TMI, but there are absolutely no precise data about the kind and degree of T wave change or how reliable an index ischemia T wave change is in general. It's certainly a subject that needs more study. Beyond question, if a patient manifested T wave change from upright to inverted during pain with a return to normal after the pain was relieved, the clinician would be justified in regarding these changes as reliable objective evidence of TMI.

What about "silent" ischemia? How often is TMI present without symptoms? With the Holter monitor and with stress testing, it's often possible to detect S-T change characteristic of ischemia in the absence of any symptoms — when the ischemia is clinically "silent." There's a great deal of current interest in silent TMI and the answers to two practical clinical questions are beginning to emerge:

1. How significant is silent myocardial ischemia? The best available data suggest that silent ischemia has exactly the same significance as symptomatic ischemia. The important fact is that ischemia is present; whether it produces symptoms or not is incidental, an accident of autonomic innervation.

2. How common is silent myocardial ischemia? Two colleagues and I published what was probably the first study in the field, in 1968 (1). We studied a large number of patients with documented coronary artery disease and recorded their symptoms at the time of acute S-T change during exercise testing. Only 41% described painful discomfort, while 46% described other symptoms such as severe abrupt dyspnea, paresthesias, or apprehension. And 10.8% reported no symptoms of any kind. Thus myocardial ischemia is either "silent" or is accompanied by symptoms other than pain in about half of all cases. A glance at Table 19-1 will aid in understanding this phenomenon: Many of the symptoms of TMI are in fact manifestations of acute, transient left heart failure.

How often does myocardial ischemia occur without ECG change? Nobody knows. One clue lies in the fact that about 20% of treadmill tests are "false negative" — that is, coronary disease is present, but there's no ECG change with exercise. Every clinician knows that the ECG often remains normal during obvious anginal pain in patients with documented coronary artery disease. There's no question, therefore, that TMI may occur without electrocardiographic change, but there are simply no data to suggest how often this occurs.

Reference

1. Phibbs B, Holmes R, Lowe C. Transient myocardial ischemia, the significance of dyspnea. Am. J. of Med. Sci. 1968; 256:210–221.

20 | Pericarditis

There are only a few specific disease entities that can be diagnosed from the ECG with a high degree of accuracy. Myocardial infarction, of course, is one. *Pericarditis* is another. Pericarditis produces an injury current on the epicardium only. The myocardium is not involved (Fig. 20-1). Because the myocardium is not involved, there are two important differences between the ECG of pericarditis and the ECG of myocardial infarction:

FIGURE 20-1
The injury current of pericarditis. Only the pericardium and occasionally the epicardium are involved. The injury current will record only an upward deflection, never a reciprocal downward deflection (except for avr, which you don't consider in this setting).

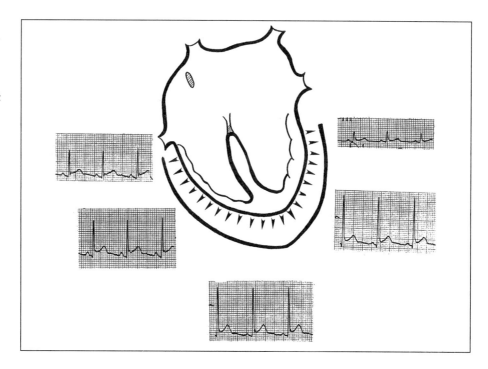

1. The S-T segments in one or more leads will be elevated. They will never be depressed. *Repeat: There is no reciprocal S-T depression in pericarditis: there is only S-T elevation.* You may see the S-T elevation in many leads or in only a few; most of the time, the S-T elevation will be widespread.

2. Since the myocardium is not involved, the QRS is not affected. There are no Q waves or other changes in the QRS complex. Changes are limited entirely to the S-T-T.

Study Figs. 20-2 and 20-3. These are typical examples of ECG deformity in pericarditis. Note the widespread S-T elevation without reciprocal depression (except in avr, where it doesn't count). As the pericarditis resolves, the S-T segments come back to baseline — usually within 72 hours. Sometimes that's all that happens. In other cases the T waves will invert progressively, moving opposite to the direction of S-T deviation, exactly as in the evolution of an infarct (Fig. 20-4). The whole evolution may take 3–5 days — a shorter time, on average, than the evolution of an infarct.

Dr. David Spodick is one of the leading investigators in this field. He pointed out a distinctive sign that often clinches the diagnosis. In acute pericarditis, the P-R segment will often show a peculiar downward displacement — an actual "downslope" as the segment approaches the

FIGURE 20-2

Typical pattern of pericarditis with S-T elevation in I, III, avf, and V3–6.

I-II-III   aVR-aVL-aVF   V1-V2-V3   V4-V5-V6

Rhythm [II] 10mm/mV

FIGURE 20-3
Pericarditis. There is obvious S-T elevation in all leads except avr, avl, and V1. Note downward deflection of P-R segment.

QRS (Fig. 20-5). This finding appears to be highly specific for acute pericarditis — the sensitivity of this particular sign has not yet been documented. In other words, when you see it, it's important evidence of pericarditis, but don't rule out pericarditis just because it's not there.

FIGURE 20-4
End stage of evolution of
pericarditis with T wave
inversion in V1–4. If you
saw only this tracing it
would be very hard to differentiate this from an anterior MI.

FIGURE 20-5
Spodick's sign. Enlarged ECG to illustrate the downward deflection of the P-R segment (arrows).

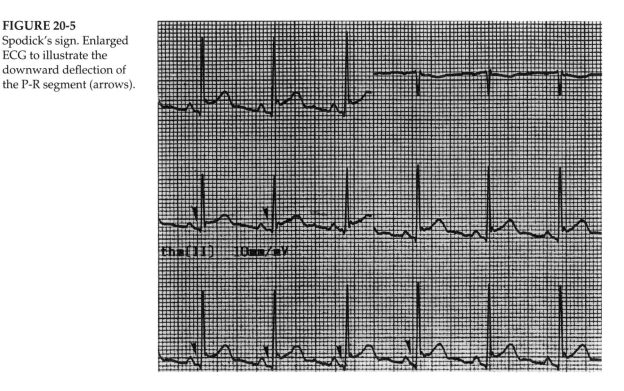

Enlargement of the Chambers of the Heart: Hypertrophy and Dilatation

Measurement of mean frontal-plane axis is important in the diagnosis of the various types of chamber enlargement. Presumably anyone reading this book knows how to calculate axis. If there's any doubt, look at Appendix II.

"Normal" Axis: Effect of Age and Body Habitus

Many texts make the statement that a "normal" axis lies between 0 and 90 degrees. This is dangerously misleading. You have to correct for age and body habitus before you decide whether an axis is normal or not.

Infants are born with a rightward axis because of high pressure in the pulmonary circuit during fetal life. An axis to the right of 100 degrees is normal in infants. The axis moves leftward during life so that an axis of 0 degrees or even slightly minus is common in adult life. Tall slender people tend to have a rightward axis because of the near-vertical position of the heart. Short stocky people commonly have a left axis because the heart tends to lie out to the left, sometimes almost horizontal. If you saw a ten-year-old with an axis of +10, you'd have to call it abnormal; the axis would be much too far to the left for a youngster of that age. If you saw an overweight 65-year-old with an axis of +90, it would be grossly abnormal. You'd look for something that would impose a load on the right heart, such as a pulmonary embolus. *Before you decide whether an axis is normal, always correct for age and body habitus.*

Chamber Enlargement

Enlargement of the chambers of the heart may be caused by dilatation or hypertrophy or both. The ventricles *dilate* when there's an increased volume of blood at the end of diastolic filling; this may be the result of valvular regurgitation or a ventricular septal defect. The ventricles *hypertrophy* when they contract against an abnormally high pressure; aortic stenosis and hypertension are of course the most common causes.

Dilatation may appear after hypertrophy when a failing heart can no longer balance inflow and outflow of blood. Many physicians do not realize that chronic ischemia can produce ventricular hypertrophy. In fact, ischemic cardiomyopathy may be the most common single cause of ventricular hypertrophy.

Atrial enlargement will always be the result of passive distension — e.g., dilatation.

For a time there was an effort to distinguish between ventricular hypertrophy and dilatation — systolic and diastolic overload — on the basis of the ECG, but that effort has been totally discarded. You can't make the distinction. In fact, the ECG is only moderately successful in detecting chamber enlargement of any kind; false-positive and false-negative readings must be expected, and the wise electrocardiographer will never be too dogmatic.

ECG Diagnosis of Atrial Enlargement

Start with the "rule of three," just as in bundle-branch block. If the P wave in the limb leads is 0.12 seconds wide or 3 mm tall, there's evidence of atrial enlargement. If the P wave is 0.12 seconds wide and *notched,* the left atrium is almost certainly enlarged. This is the classic "P-mitrale" so named by the French because it appears most commonly with the large left atrium of mitral disease (Fig. 21-1A). The P-mitrale will most commonly be seen in II and III. If the P waves in II, III, and avf are 3 mm tall and peaked (the "gothic" P, because it's supposed to look like a cathedral), the right atrium is enlarged. This is commonly called "P-pulmonale" because it's most commonly seen with severe lung disease accompanied by pulmonary hypertension (Fig. 21-1B). Some writ-

FIGURE 21-1
(A) Left atrial enlargement, as reflected in the limb leads. (B) Right atrial enlargement, as reflected in the limb leads.

A

B

FIGURE 21-2
Normal diphasic P in V1. Note that the P wave consists of a small upward deflection followed by a small negative deflection. These deflections represent right atrial and left atrial activation, respectively.

FIGURE 21-3
(A) Left atrial enlargement, reflected in the deep negative component of P in V1. In this strip, the enlarged left atrium is posterior. There is a large negative P wave in V1 because the wave activating the left atrium is moving *away from* V1. The negative P wave must enclose at least 1 mm^2 to be significant. (B) Right atrial enlargement, reflected in a tall, wide, positive component of P in V1. The right atrium is anterior. The large P wave is positive in V1 because the wave activating the right atrium is moving *toward* V1. The positive P wave must also enclose at least 1 mm^2 to be significant.

ers pick the number 2.5 in the diagnosis of atrial enlargement — thus if the P wave is 0.10 seconds wide or 2.5 mm tall, they read hypertrophy. I prefer to be more specific even though possibly less sensitive, hence the criteria outlined above.

The P wave in V1 can also be helpful. Think of the right atrium as the anterior atrium and the left as the posterior. Look closely at P-V1 in most ECGs and you'll see a small upward deflection followed by a small negative deflection (Fig. 21-2). Since the right atrium is anterior, the wave activating it moves *toward* V1, producing the upward deflection. By the same token, since the left atrium is posterior, the wave activating it moves *away* from V1 and produces a negative deflection. If either the positive or negative components of the P wave enclose an area equal to a generous square millimeter, there's evidence of atrial abnormality — either enlargement or slow conduction through a diseased syncytium (Fig. 21-3A and B).

ECG Diagnosis of Left Ventricular Hypertrophy (LVH)

The diagnosis of hypertrophy of ventricular musculature is based on a few simple concepts:

1. The thicker the heart muscle, the taller the R wave it produces. Thus an abnormally tall R is one of the important criteria of hypertrophy. Obviously, an abnormally tall R on one side of the electric field of the heart means that there'll be an abnormally deep S on the opposite side. Excessive voltage, positive or negative, is therefore the key criterion for hypertrophy (Fig. 21–4).

2. The mean electric axis will swing toward the thickest mass of myocardium. If the left ventricle is enlarged, the mean axis will swing leftward. (Correspondingly, of course, right ventricular hypertrophy will move the axis to the right.)

3. A peculiar S-T-T configuration may appear in leads over the hypertrophied ventricle. The S-T segment is depressed and downsloping and the T wave is inverted in a "hockey stick" configuration with a low, slow descent and a rapid upstroke (Fig. 21-5).

FIGURE 21-4
Increased voltage in left ventricular hypertrophy.

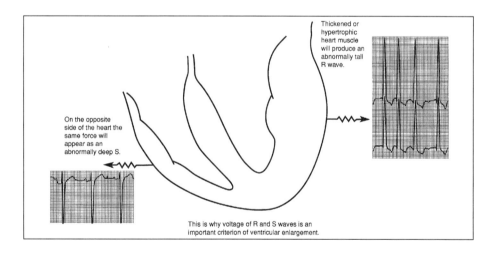

Thickened or hypertrophic heart muscle will produce an abnormally tall R wave.

On the opposite side of the heart the same force will appear as an abnormally deep S.

This is why voltage of R and S waves is an important criterion of ventricular enlargement.

FIGURE 21-5
S-T-T "strain" pattern in left ventricular hypertrophy.

4. Left atrial enlargement. Since the mitral valve is open all through diastole, increased LV pressures will be transmitted back to the left atrium, with subsequent left atrial enlargement. In the absence of mitral disease, left atrial enlargement is a fairly reliable reflection of the pathophysiology that has produced left ventricular enlargement and failure.

5. Delayed onset of instrinsicoid deflection. The thicker the myocardium, the longer it takes for the activating wave to traverse it. When the myocardium is abnormally thickened, therefore, it takes longer than normal for the R wave to complete its rise from base to peak. This time interval has the clumsy title of "time of onset of intrinsicoid deflection." The intrinsicoid deflection is defined as the time to the beginning of the rapid fall from the peak of the R. (A more logical term would be "R wave inscription time," but medical jargonists will never settle for a simple term if they can come up with something more complicated.) Normal value is less than .05 seconds.

Now you can put these elements together into a system for diagnosing left ventricular hypertrophy. The most authoritative correlation of these five variables was accomplished by Romhilt and Estes (1). These investigators measured postmortem wall thickness and ventricular mass as their basis for comparison. They produced a point-score system reproduced in Table 21-1. Note that in this system, "increased voltage" means 30 mm in a precordial lead and 20 mm in a limb lead. This point-score system still gives the best correlation with left ventricular hypertrophy.

An older study by Sokolow and Lyons (2) was carried on before the days of catheterization or echocardiograms and the authors did not use postmortem measurements as their basis of comparison. They simply compared patients with and without hypertension on the assumption that hypertensive patients were more likely to have left ventricular hypertrophy. On this tenuous basis they concluded that if the sum of the S wave in V2 and the R in V5 equaled 35 mm, left ventricular hypertrophy was likely to be present. Other studies subsequently added voltage in avl greater than 11 mm as a criterion of LVH. These voltage criteria are widely used today, and it's worthwhile examining their accuracy.

Cumming and Proudfit (3) tested these voltage criteria against postmortem findings and found that if the criterion of the sum of R V5 and S V2 was applied there were 39% false-positive readings. In other words, the voltage criteria of Sokolow and Lyons indicated LVH when the heart was in fact normal about 40% of the time. Increased voltage in avl was similarly inaccurate: False-positive readings equaled about 36%. If increased precordial voltage was combined with increased voltage in avl,

Table 21-1. The Romhilt-Estes point-score for detection of left ventricular hypertrophy

1. Voltage. Any of the following: R or S wave in limb leads, 20 mm; S V1–V2, 30 mm, R V5–V6, 30 mm. 3 points.
2. S-T-T deformity of "strain" type: 2 points.
3. Left atrial enlargement: 3 points.*
4. Left axis, 30 or greater: 2 points.
5. QRS duration 0.09 or greater (less than 0.12): 1 point.**
6. R wave inscription time in V5, V6 = 0.05 seconds or more: 1 point.
7. Left ventricular hypertrophy: 5 points.
8. Probable left ventricular hypertrophy: 4 points.

*"Left axis" should mean axis in the –20 to –30 range. Extreme left axis of –40 or higher means that there is a conduction defect in the left ventricle (anterior fascicular block) and such an axis cannot be used to establish presence of LVH.
**"QRS" duration of 0.09 or greater applies only if the widening is less than 0.11–0.12 — that is, if the widening is not caused by bundle-branch block.
Source: Romhilt DW and Estes EH. Point-score system for the ECG diagnosis of left ventricular hypertrophy. *Am. Heart J.* 1968;75:752.

the accuracy was improved, although the design of this study precluded an exact percentage.

Reicheck and Devereux (4) carried out a precise study correlating ECG criteria for LVH with postmortem findings. Their conclusions are worth repeating:

1. In a clinical population with a moderate incidence of LVH, both Romhilt-Estes and Sokolow-Lyons voltage criteria are highly specific: When present, they indicate LVH with about 95% confidence.

2. Neither set of criteria is acceptably sensitive: The fact that these criteria are *not* fulfilled doesn't mean that LVH isn't present. With Romhilt-Estes criteria, sensitivity is only 50%, whereas with Sokolow-Lyons it is 21%. In other words, a normal ECG doesn't rule out LVH. With the best current criteria the ECG will miss the diagnosis about half the time.

3. In a population with a low prevalence of LVH (less than 10%), there will be more false-positive than true-positive readings. In other words, the ECG will give a false reading of LVH in this group more often than a true one. The moral here is that the physician reading ECGs for routine physical examinations or for life-insurance applications should not diagnose LVH from the ECG alone. This is especially true when only voltage criteria are present.

FIGURE 21-6
Left ventricular hypertrophy with all the elements of the Romhilt-Estes system: voltage, axis, "strain" S-T-T pattern, left atrial enlargement, and delay of onset of intrinsicoid deflection.

Figure 21-6 illustrates many of the criteria for LVH.

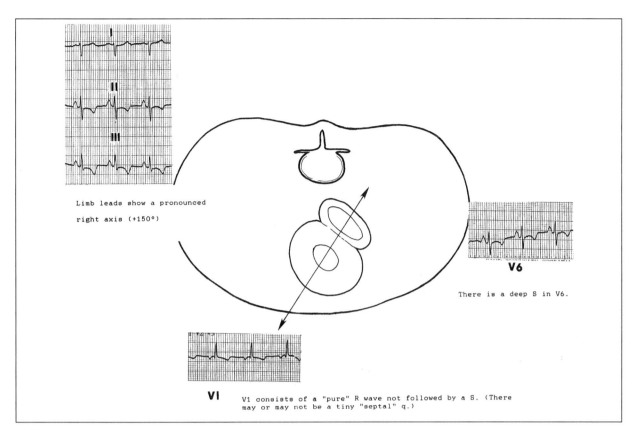

Limb leads show a pronounced

right axis (+150°)

V6

There is a deep S in V6.

V1

V1 consists of a "pure" R wave not followed by a S. (There may or may not be a tiny "septal" q.)

FIGURE 21-7
Anatomy and ECG of Type A RVH. There is extreme elevation of RV pressure, as in pulmonic stenosis or severe pulmonary hypertension. RV forces are larger than LV forces throughout depolarization. If pulmonary hypertension is the cause, the PA pressure will be at least two-thirds of systemic.

ECG Diagnosis of Right Ventricular Hypertrophy (RVH)
Here the ECG correlation is probably better than it is with LVH. The classification of Chou and Helm (5) is very useful.

1. Type A RVH. This is a very simple diagnosis. V1 consists of a simple R wave and hence looks like the letter "A." There's an extreme right axis (Fig. 21-7). This is the most severe type of RVH. The type A pattern means that the pressure in the right heart is extremely high — at least two-thirds of systemic pressure. The PA systolic pressure will be in the range of 85 mm Hg or higher. It's the kind of RVH you would expect with pulmonic stenosis or with severe congenital left-to-right shunts. Figure 21-8 is a typical example of Type A RVH.

FIGURE 21-8
Typical ECG of Type A
RVH, reflecting extremely
high PA-RV pressures.

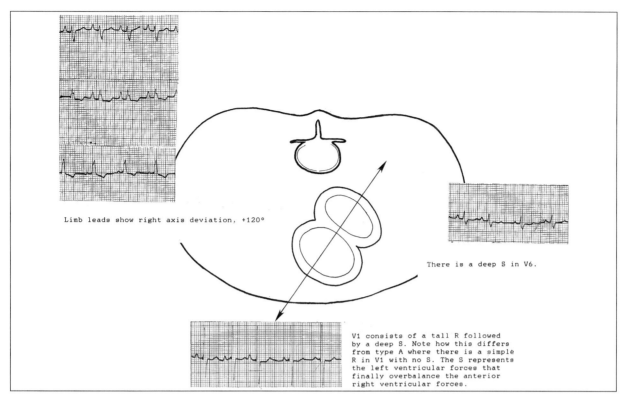

Limb leads show right axis deviation, +120°

There is a deep S in V6.

V1 consists of a tall R followed by a deep S. Note how this differs from type A where there is a simple R in V1 with no S. The S represents the left ventricular forces that finally overbalance the anterior right ventricular forces.

FIGURE 21-9
Anatomy and ECG of Type B RVH. This is the pattern seen with moderate right ventricular hypertrophy. Mitral stenosis with pulmonary artery pressure of 60/40 would be a typical example. Right ventricular forces dominate initially, but left ventricular activation finally pulls the forces of depolarization back and to the left.

2. Type B RVH. This connotes a less severe type of RVH than Type A. V1 consists of an initial tall R followed by an S. The R will be at least equal to the S. This terminal S in V1 is the important distinction between Type A and Type B. There will be a right axis in the frontal-place leads (Fig. 21-9). Type B RVH appears with moderate elevation of PA and right-heart pressures — a PA pressure of 60/40, for example. It's the kind of pattern you often see with mitral stenosis. Figure 21-10 is a typical example of Type B RVH.

FIGURE 21-10
Typical Type B RVH associated with moderate elevation of PA-RV pressures.

Across the entire precordium there
is an almost identical pattern of
a small r followed by a deep S.
This combination is always seen with
severe chronic obstructive pulmonary
disease chiefly of the predominant
emphysema or "pink puffer" type.
It represents one of the most specific
correlations in electrocardiography.

FIGURE 21-11
Anatomy and ECG of Type C RVH. This is a curious and highly specific pattern. The axis in the limb leads is "so far right that it's left." In other words, it's about +240 degrees, as shown in the diagram. This is sometimes called the S1-S2-S3 pattern in the limb leads; it has also been termed "axis illusion" and "pseudo-left axis."

3. Type C RVH. This is the most specific pattern in terms of correlation with disease. Careful correlative studies by Dr. Carl Schmock and his colleagues at the University of Colorado proved that this occurs exclusively with chronic obstructive lung disease, predominantly in the "pink puffer" subgroup, where the principal pathology consists of hyperdistension of terminal bronchioles and alveoli. Leads I, II, and III are all negative — in other words, there's a dominant S in I, II, and III. The frontal axis is therefore in the quadrant between –90 and –180. The axis is in fact so far to the right that it's left. This is called "axis illusion" or "pseudo-left axis." The precordial leads consist exclusively of a small r with a deep S in every lead from V1 to V6 (Fig. 21-11). This pattern is amazingly specific. When you see it, diagnose the type of chronic obstructive lung disease associated with predominant emphysema with complete confidence (Fig. 21-12).

FIGURE 21-12
Typical Type C RVH associated with severe COPD.

References

1. Romhilt DW and Estes EH. Point-score system for the ECG diagnosis of left ventricular hypertrophy. *Am. Heart J.* 1968; 75:752.
2. Sokolow M and Lyons TP. Ventricular complex in left ventricular hypertrophy as obtained by unipolar precordial and limb leads. *Am. Heart J.* 1949; 37:161.
3. Cumming G and Proudfit W. High-voltage QRS complexes in the absence of left ventricular hypertrophy. *Circulation* 1959; XIX:406–409.
4. Reicheck R and Devereux M. Left ventricular hypertrophy: relationship to anatomic, echocardiographic and electrocardiographic findings. *Circulation* 1981; 63:1391.
5. Chou T and Helm R. *Clinical vectorcardiography.* New York: Grune and Stratton, 1967; 77–99.

22

"Nonspecific" Myocardial Pathology

It's time to consider limitations. It's safe to say that about 75% of all ECG abnormalities do not fall into any of the specific disease categories described in the last three chapters. The honest electrocardiographer will recognize the limitations of the ECG and will use the term "nonspecific" many times a day. Properly interpreted, this means that the ECG is recording the presence of some kind of myocardial pathology. The term means further that it's not possible to say what kind of pathology is present or how severe it is. Don't try. Restraint and modesty are the hallmarks of the competent electrocardiographer; a special kind of medicolegal and diagnostic Hell awaits those who "overread."

A great many diseases and toxins can attack the myocardium, all with the same unfortunate outcome: myocardial cells die and are replaced by scar tissue. These changes may be reflected in the ECG, and when they are, they'll appear as "nonspecific" abnormalities.

Coronary artery disease can cause diffuse myocardial scarring even though there has never been an actual infarct. A postmortem on any patient with prolonged angina pectoris will always reveal many small areas of scarring scattered throughout the heart muscle. This is the basis of "ischemic cardiomyopathy." Sometimes there will even be localized masses of scar tissue — the phenomenon Dr. Hurst referred to as "hunk disease" because there's a "hunk" of scar tissue that formed quietly, without infarction.

Viral infections, including AIDS, lupus erythematosus, polyarteritis nodosa, sarcoidosis, scleroderma; drugs like cocaine; and toxins like beryllium can all leave scarred, nonfunctioning myocardium. In addition there's a substantial group of patients who turn up with evidence of cardiomyopathy for no discernible reason—the "idiopathic" cardiomyopathies.

There are no specific ECG patterns in this group of diseases. You'll see changes in the ECG that permit you to make the diagnosis of "myocardial pathology" and at that point you put down the dictating machine and stop.

ECG Diagnosis

Most of the time these changes will be in the T waves. You've already learned about the "specific" patterns of S-T-T deformity in myocardial infarction, pericarditis, and hypertrophy. It's time to learn the rules about "nonspecific" T wave deformity.

The T waves should be upright in *most* leads. A flat, diphasic, or inverted T wave is abnormal in *most* leads. Note that we said "most," not "all." There are some leads where it's normal to see inverted T waves. Normal individuals will always have inverted T waves in avr. They may have inverted T waves in lead III and in V1 or V2 (Fig. 22-1). When you see diphasic or inverted T waves without QRS or T wave change in any other leads, the reading is "nonspecific T wave deformity consistent with myocardial pathology." Stop right there. That's all you can say.

This is a very sound set of rules based on observation of millions of ECGs by every qualified observer in the field. For an intelligent physi-

FIGURE 22-1
Leads in which an inverted T wave is a normal finding.

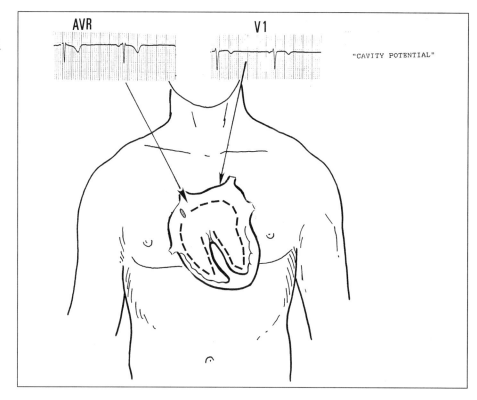

cian, that's not enough. It's necessary to know why it's normal to have
deformed T waves in some leads and not in others.

Look at Fig. 22-2. This explains the inverted T waves in avr and sometimes in V1 and V2. Think of the inside, or "cavity," of the heart as negatively charged. When you float an electrode into the superior vena
cava, for instance, all deflections will be negative because you'll be
recording from the negatively charged "cavity" of the heart. To put it another way, all the activating waves are moving away from the recording
electrode because of its position above the heart. Avr always "looks
down" into the cavity of the heart, hence the negative deflections. V1
and V2 can record the same kind of cavity potential, depending on the
position of the heart in the chest.

How about lead III? This trips up many cardiologists, so it should be
explained at some length. In about 15% of normal individuals you'll see
a significant Q wave in lead III. You'll see inverted T waves in about the
same percentage of normals, and often you'll see the Q and the inverted
T together — a combination that has created many an imaginary infarct.

The simplest way to find whether a Q or an inverted T in III mean anything is to look at avf. If you don't see these deflections in avf, forget

them. They're a normal variant that appears only in lead III. Why only in lead III? Think about how leads I, II, and III are set up. They're bipolar leads, which means that they measure the difference in potential between two points. They're like the simple galvanometer you set up in high-school physics with a positive pole and a negative pole. Lead III is set up to measure the difference in potential between the left leg (avf) and the left arm (avl). The left leg is the "positive" electrode. This means that when the left leg is positive *compared to the left arm* there will be an upward deflection in lead III. When the left leg is negative *compared to the left arm* there will be a downward deflection in lead III. Remember that in a bipolar system, "negative" can simply mean "less positive." Thus if avf is registering a force of 1 mm while avl is registering a force of 4 mm, there will be a downward deflection in III — not because there's any real negativity anywhere but simply because the left leg is recording a smaller positive potential than the left arm. In other words, lead III equals avf – avl or +1 – (+4) = –3. You're looking at "signed numbers" just as you did in the fifth grade. *Whenever the T in avl is larger than the T in avf there will be an inverted T III even though T avf and T avl are both positive.* Figures 22-3 and 22-4 illustrate this simple point.

FIGURE 22-3
A "physiologic" inverted T III. T avf is flat while T avl is large and upright. Lead III equals the electric difference between avf and avl. In other words you derive T III by subtracting T avl from T avf. T avf is flat while T avl encloses an area of about 4.5 mm². When you subtract 4.5 from 0 you get a –4.5, that is, a negative T in III. All the negative T III means is that the T in avl is larger than the T in avf.

FIGURE 22-4
Same phenomenon. T avf is small — about 1.5 mm² in area. T avl is much larger, about 4 mm². Subtracting avl from avf leaves you with a negative T III even though the actual T potentials at both the left leg and left arm are positive.

You won't see this effect in leads I or II because the indifferent electrode is the right arm, or avr, where everything is negative. There's no positive potential to subtract as there is in avl. That's why you see this curious effect only in lead III.

For the same reason, a Q in III doesn't mean anything unless you also see it in avf. In Fig. 22-5 you'll note that the initial part of the QRS is a tiny "septal" q, followed by a small, slurred, slowly rising r. In avl, on the other hand, there's a sharply rising R. In other words, avl is positive compared to avf all through the first half of the QRS. Lead III obediently records a downward deflection all this time — hence the deep Q that doesn't mean anything. All it's telling you is that there's a stronger positive potential at the left arm than at the left leg all through the first part of depolarization. This is of course a normal variant and that's why you'll see wide Q waves in 15% of normal individuals.

You may ask, "Why bother to record the bipolar limb leads at all? Why not just record avr, avl, and avf, since those are the actual isolated potentials at the right shoulder, left shoulder, and left leg?" Good question. The augmented unipolar limb leads contain all the information you need and we go on recording I, II, and III out of habit.

FIGURE 22-5
The "physiologic Q" of lead III. Avf records a small initial R while avl records a tall one. Lead III records a negative deflection or Q wave until the potential in avl falls below the potential in avf in the last part of the QRS. Moral: When you see a Q III always look at avf to see what caused it.

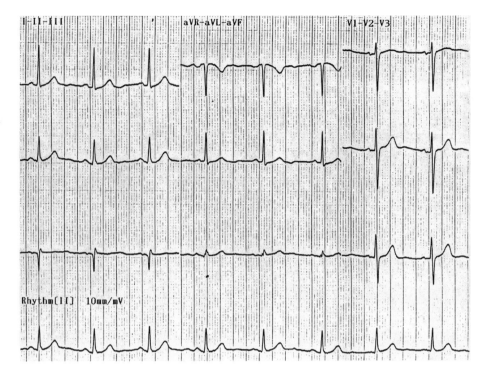

Figures 22-6 through 22-11 are examples of "nonspecific" T wave deformity. Obviously, the various types of cardiac pathology can affect the ventricular conducting network and any kind of intraventricular delay may appear. There are some statistical associations — for example, in Chagas's cardiomyopathy, right bundle-branch block is common — but, overall, delay in intraventricular conduction must be classed as a "nonspecific" finding that may be a result of anything from ischemic cardiomyopathy to leishmaniasis. Look outside the ECG for specific causes!

FIGURE 22-6

Diffuse T wave deformity in lateral, inferior, and anterior leads. Note the change in ST-T-T morphology with the premature atrial beats in V1–3. You're seeing a kind of one-beat stress test with more deformity at a more rapid rate. The symmetrical inversion of the T waves suggests a "coronary" configuration, but it's only suggestive, not diagnostic.

Rhythm [II] 10mm/mV

FIGURE 22-7
Proper diagnosis: "anterior and lateral S-T-T deformity consistent with myocardial pathology." Period. End of diagnosis.

I-II-III   aVR-aVL-aVF   V1-V2-V3   V4-V5-V6

Rhythm [II] 10mm/mV

FIGURE 22-8
Some of the criteria of
LVH are here — increased
voltage, left axis, "hockey
stick" S-T-T. Diagnosis:
"some criteria for left ventricular hypertrophy. S-T-T
deformity may be the re-
sult of hypertrophy, ischemia, or both."

I-II-III   aVR-aVl-aVF   V1-V2-V3   V4-V5-V6

Sinus rhythm; Rate 70, PR 17, QRS 08, wide notch P2,3 AVF flattened TV4,5,6.
some diffuse lateral T-wave flattening. Evidence of left atrial enlargement.
NO acute change.

Rhythm [II] 10mm/mV

FIGURE 22-9
Diffuse T wave flattening in lateral, inferior, and anterolateral leads. A flat T wave in one lead may not be significant, but diffuse T wave flattening in two or more lead systems is always significant and may be the result of myocardial pathology. It might also be the result of extracardiac metabolic or toxic factors.

FIGURE 22-10
Diagnosis: "abnormal tracing. Right axis deviation. Inferolateral S-T-T deformity consistent with myocardial pathology."

I-II-III   aVR-aVl-aVF   V1-V2-V3   V4-V5-V6

Rhythm [II] 10mm/mV

FIGURE 22-11
Diagnosis: "diffuse S-T-T deformity with S-T depression in inferior and lateral leads, T wave inversion V3–4. Findings consistent with myocardial pathology."

23

Electrolytes and Drugs

Electrolytes

Changes in the levels of serum calcium and potassium can affect the electrocardiogram. Think of calcium as the "energizer" of the heart. After all, it is the movement of calcium into the myocardial cells that begins the chemistry of contraction. With an elevated serum calcium, the Q-T interval is shortened. In other words, with a high level of calcium, the heart is activated more quickly than normal (Fig. 23-1).

Hypocalcemia has exactly the opposite effect: The Q-T interval is prolonged (Fig. 23-2). Note that the prolongation is in the S-T segment, not in the T wave. This is an important point when differentiating quinidine effect from hypocalcemia.

Potassium has been described as the "soothing syrup" of the heart. Too much of it puts all the pacemaking and conducting tissues to sleep. Hyperkalemia depresses AV and IV conduction and, in higher levels, can completely suppress the sinus node. There are progressive levels of

FIGURE 23-1
Hypercalcemia. Q-T interval, 0.21 seconds.

I-II-III   aVR-aVL-aVF   V1-V2-V3   V4-V5-V6

Rhythm [II] 10mm/mV

303

FIGURE 23-2
Hypocalcemia. Q-T interval, 0.56 seconds.

FIGURE 23-3
Hyperpotassemia, moderate. Note tall, peaked T waves in V2, 3, and 4. (Rule of thumb: A tall, peaked T becomes significant when it's more than half the amplitude of the R in a lead that consists entirely of an R.)

FIGURE 23-4
More severe elevation of K. Prolonged P-R interval and giant, peaked T waves.

FIGURE 23-5
Serum K of 8.8 meq/L.
Prolonged P-R, widened
QRS, peaked T waves.

FIGURE 23-6
Dangerous elevation of K
at 10 meq/L; extremely
slow IV conduction with
QRS of 0.25 seconds.

FIGURE 23-7
Dangerous elevation of K,
over 10 meq/L; P-R 0.26,
QRS 0.26. Obvious ex-
treme delay in intraven-
tricular conduction.

FIGURE 23-8
K in excess of 10 meq/L;
complete suppression of
sinus node activity. The
junctional rhythm is lifesaving.

change, depending on the level of serum potassium. Moderate elevation
of K produces tall, peaked T waves (Figs. 23-3 and 23-4). Severe elevation of K causes depression of conduction in the bundle-branch system.
Various types of QRS prolongation appear as serum K reaches levels of
8 to 9 meq/L (Figs. 23-5, 23-6, and 23-7). With very severe elevation of K,
there may be depression of sinus node function. The P waves become
sparse or actually disappear. Life is maintained by idiojunctional or idioventricular rhythms (Fig. 23-8). Lethal elevation of K at levels around
12 meq/L are likely to produce ventricular fibrillation or standstill.

Hypokalemia produces depression of the S-T segment similar to digitalis effect. There are also prominent U waves. The giant U waves often merge with the T waves to give an illusion of a prolonged Q-T, but this is an artifact: In fact the Q-T interval doesn't change (Fig. 23-9).

Drugs

The digitalis-toxic arrhythmias have been described in Chapter 16. They're so common, so dangerous, and so specific in terms of treatment that they deserve a chapter of their own. Digitalis compounds commonly cause depression of the S-T segments with the "wet-noodle" bowing as illustrated in Figs. 23-10, 23-11, and 23-12. This kind of S-T

FIGURE 23-9
Severe hypokalemia, 2.1 meq/L. There is striking S-T depression, resembling digitalis effect. Prominent U waves give a false impression of prolongation of Q-T.

FIGURE 23-10
Typical sagging of S-T segments seen in practically all patients taking digitalis for any length of time.

FIGURE 23-11
Digitalis effect striking
S-T-T deformity, with T
waves "swallowed up" in
the depressed S-T seg-
ments.

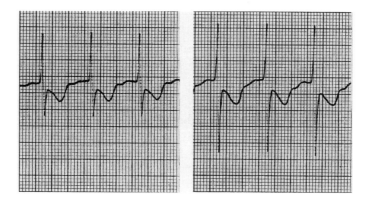

FIGURE 23-12
A combination of digitalis
effect (the sagging S-T segments) with digitalis *toxicity* (the accelerated
junctional rhythm with
complete AV dissociation).

depression is *not* a sign of digitalis toxicity; it should be described only as "digitalis effect." Minimal prolongation of the P-R is common with digitalis therapy. Like S-T depression it should be described only as "digitalis effect," not as digitalis toxicity. If you see a fixed P-R of 0.22 to 0.24 seconds, it doesn't mean you have to discontinue digitalis.

Quinidine

Quinidine has a straightforward effect: it's a depressant. It depresses impulse formation and conduction everywhere in the heart. In the AV node there's a diphasic effect. In small doses quinidine opposes the vagus and accelerates AV nodal conduction; in the presence of atrial fibrillation or flutter there may be an increase in ventricular rate with quinidine. Quinidine sometimes leads to 1:1 conduction in the presence of flutter with dangerous results, but the vagolytic effect is minor in this setting. The real problem with quinidine in flutter is that it slows the flutter rate in the atria so that every atrial impulse is conducted to the ventricles. Look at the flutter rate next time you give a patient quinidine and you'll see for yourself: The atrial rate may slow from 300 to 215 or thereabouts. In higher concentrations, quinidine depresses AV nodal conduction and can produce any kind of AV nodal block.

The most common ECG manifestation of quinidine effect is prolongation of the Q-T interval. There is almost always some prolongation of

FIGURE 23-13
Minimal quinidine effect on Q-T interval. The interval is approximately 0.4 seconds, which is prolonged for a rate of 93. This degree of prolongation is very common and is not a reason to discontinue the drug. Quinidine can produce "sagging" of the S-T segment that looks exactly like digitalis effect.

FIGURE 23-14
Pronounced quinidine effect with Q-T interval of 0.54 seconds, at a rate of 86. Note the depressed S-T segments. Part of the large wave that runs all the way to the next P may be a U wave incorporated in the T.

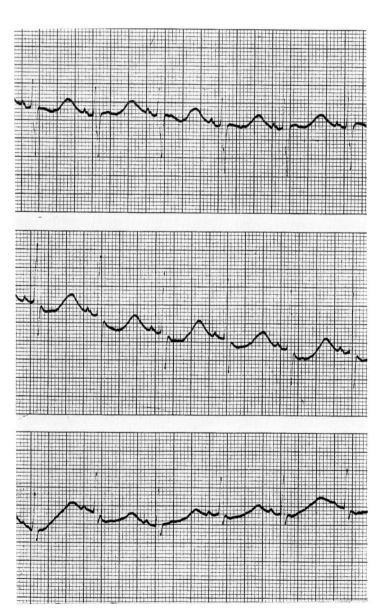

Q-T with therapeutic levels of quinidine, and this is not per se an indication to stop the drug (Fig. 23-13). Extreme prolongation of Q-T, however, increases the danger of torsade: In fact, it's likely that this is the sole significant basis for the cardiac toxicity of quinidine (Fig. 23-14). The word *extreme* cannot be defined precisely at this time, but a reasonable rough guess would be that any Q-T prolongation more than 25% above the calculated maximum for age and sex presents a real hazard; the drug should probably be discontinued. Quinidine depresses the cells in the bundle-branch system and delays intraventricular conduction. If quinidine causes widening of the QRS to more than 15% above baseline, the drug should be stopped.

It's customary to warn about giving the drug to patients with bundle-branch block for fear that conduction in the other bundle branch might fail. This is a warning that probably has no basis in fact. In fifty years of administering quinidine, I have never seen serious depression of intraventricular conduction. I suppose it happens, but it's very, very rare. I can't remember the last time I saw significant QRS widening caused by quinidine, and all current studies bear this out. This particular hazard has been grossly exaggerated: The presence of bundle-branch block or other intraventricular conduction defect is not a contraindication to the use of quinidine. The real hazard with quinidine, to reiterate, is Q-T prolongation leading to torsade. Other 1A drugs, such as procaine amide and disopyramide, can prolong the Q-T interval, with the attendant danger of torsade.

Tricyclic Antidepressants
Any drug in this category can depress conduction within the ventricles. Nonspecific widening of the QRS, frank bundle-branch block, or AV block caused by failure of both bundle branches can result. Like quinidine, these drugs can also affect AV nodal conduction, producing any variety of AV nodal block, although this is less common than delay in the bundle-branch system.

Phenothiazines
The phenothiazines as a group have effects much like quinidine: prolongation of Q-T interval and depression of conduction within the ventricles. AV block has occasionally occurred with overdoses of these drugs. Sudden death in apparently healthy individuals taking these drugs is doubtless the result of torsade following Q-T prolongation.

24

Two Special Cases: Pulmonary Emboli and Hypothermia

Pulmonary Emboli

The most important thing to remember about pulmonary emboli is that most of them have no effect on the ECG at all. Never rule out a pulmonary embolus just because the ECG remains normal! The reason for this is obvious: The lungs have such an abundant blood supply that an embolus must compromise a really major segment of the lung before it has any effect on pressure in the pulmonary artery. An embolus that compromises a large segment of a lung can create high pressures in the pulmonary artery and in the right heart. The ECG will reflect that sudden rise in pressure in the lesser circulation. The changes are quite predictable:

1. There will be a sudden swing of the axis to the right, often with a deep S in I. A small septal q will usually be present in III, which gave rise to the old "SI-Q-III" combination you still read about in textbooks. That phrase is a hangover from the primitive days in electrocardiography when we had only leads I, II, and III and didn't really know what a septal q was. The simple fact is that the sudden rise in PA and RV pressures swings the axis rightward, just as you'd expect; whether there's a small q in III is irrelevant.

2. There may be an incomplete right bundle-branch block pattern. This is usually seen in more extreme cases with significant elevation of PA-RV pressures. This will be accompanied by a right axis of the initial forces (Fig. 24-1).

3. There may be a peculiar type of S-T depression in the limb leads. There is a horizontal depression of the S-T with an abrupt, almost vertical rise into the T. The shape of the S-T-T complex gave rise to the German term of "Treppe" or "steps," and in fact the S-T-T complex does resemble a staircase. This peculiar configuration is rarely seen in any other setting. In other words, it's not at all sensitive, but it's very spe-

FIGURE 24-1
Incomplete right bundle-branch block with rightward axis of initial forces in the limb leads. This is a typical configuration seen with a massive pulmonary embolus.

cific. In Fig. 24-2 there is a typical example of the "Treppe" type of S-T-T deformity combined with a right axis that had appeared abruptly at the time of symptoms. This was a major pulmonary embolus with a fatal outcome.

Pulmonary emboli can also produce S-T-T deformities of the "nonspecific" variety described in Chap. 22.

Hypothermia

There is one specific deformity associated with hypothermia: a deflection of the late forces of the QRS called an "Osborne wave." A wide, slurred deflection appears at the end of the downstroke of the R (Fig. 24-3). This is a relatively mild example; sometimes an Osborne wave can be enormous, constituting most of the ventricular complex.

FIGURE 24-2
Classic findings with a pulmonary embolus. A deep S has appeared in lead I, and there's a small septal q in III. The sharp angle where the depressed S-T joins the T in I and avl is the typical "Treppe" or "staircase" deformity.

FIGURE 24-3
The Osborne wave of hypothermia. These are leads V2–5. The wide, slurred terminal portion of the R is the characteristic deformity of hypothermia.

Self-Assessment III

FIGURE III-1

1. A physician calls for help. He's been treating this patient's chronic atrial fibrillation with digoxin, but he notes that the pulse has become more rapid and the patient is in distress. Giving more digoxin only seems to make it worse. Cause? Treatment?

FIGURE III-2   2. Diagnosis? Number of criteria to support the diagnosis?

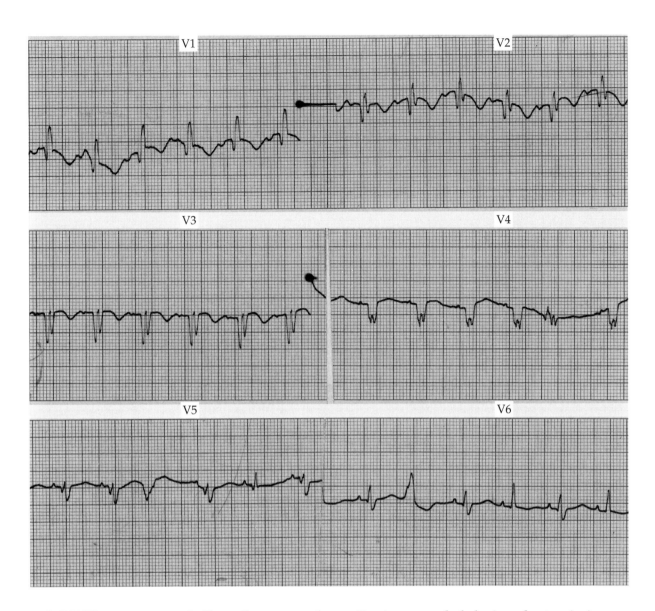

FIGURE III-3

3. Two diagnoses, please. Tracing recorded during chest pain in a patient who had a normal ECG a month ago. Prognosis? What's happening in V6?

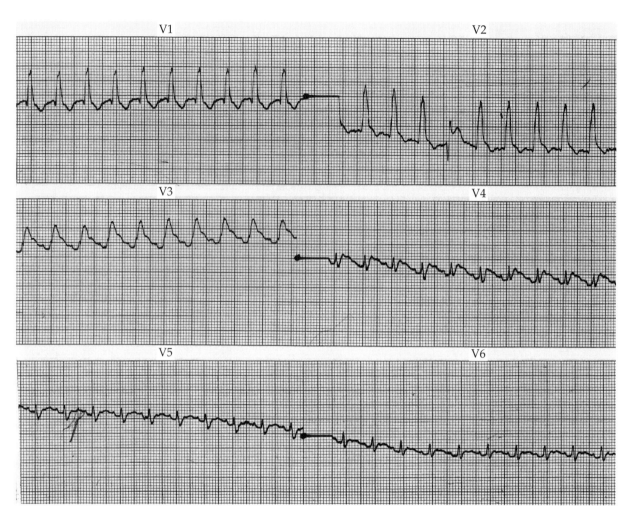

FIGURE III-4

4. Tracing handed to you from the emergency room. Two diagnoses and proof?

A

FIGURE III-5A and B   5. The patient had a normal ECG with normal axis two weeks ago. Diagnosis? How supported? Additional feature?

B

FIGURE III-6   6. Leads V1, 2, and 3. Wide beats followed by narrow beats. Diagnosis?

FIGURE III-7

7. Two diagnoses. Proof?

FIGURE III-8

8. Just from this rhythm strip, what symptoms would you anticipate? What clinical diagnosis? What cause would you rule out as a first step in treatment?

FIGURE III-9

9. What statement can you make about this ECG? What statement(s) can you not make?

I

III

AVR   AVL   AVF

V1   V2

V3   V4

V5   V6

FIGURE III-10   10. Complete diagnosis? Possible causes?

FIGURE III-11

11. Rapid rhythm; bizarre, changing QRST morphology. Two diagnoses, please (each a matter of life or death here).

FIGURE III-12

12. This rhythm strip pops up in the CCU. What danger confronts this patient? Probable cause? Treatment?

FIGURE III-13

13. This calls for tough reasoning. There's an obvious diagnosis here,

but you have to use deductive logic to find it. Cause of the arrhythmia? Source of the P waves? State of AV conduction? Clinical entity?

FIGURE III-14A

14. What hemodynamic prediction can you make from this tracing? What pathology of what chambers?

FIGURE III-14B

FIGURE III-15   15. Complete diagnosis? With what confidence? Why?

FIGURE III-16   16. Complete diagnosis? With what confidence? Why?

FIGURE III-17

17. This tracing came over the telephone transmitter from a remote hospital's CCU. Mechanism? Cause of pauses? State of AV conduction?

FIGURE III-18

18. Wide-beat tachycardia. Precise diagnosis? Significance?

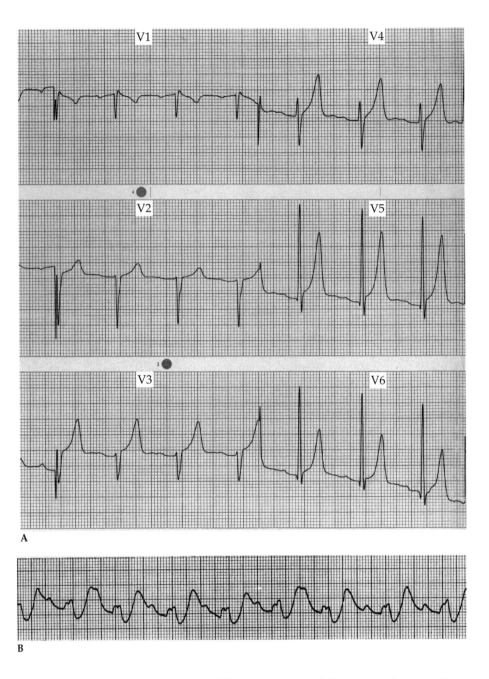

A

B

FIGURE III-19 19. Tracings A and B illustrate different stages of the same abnormality.

FIGURE III-20

20. Just to keep you honest: narrow beats and wide beats. Cause of the two wide beats?

FIGURE III-21

21. Here's a test of your powers of observation. This specific arrhythmia isn't described in the text. What do you see? (Rare and dangerous.)

FIGURE III-22

22. This arrhythmia appeared on the monitor in CCU. The patient had been admitted with a diagnosis of "probable anterior MI." Rhythm? Morphologic change? Significance?

FIGURE III-23

23. Rhythm strip in the ER. Diagnosis? Possibility or probability of special pathophysiology? Steps to clarify? Treatment?

FIGURE III-24

24. The asymptomatic patient was told she had had a previous inferior MI on the basis of this tracing. Comment?

Answers

1. The periods of regular rhythm, rate 152, obviously represent runs of junctional tachycardia interrupting atrial fibrillation. This is one of the most common manifestations of digitalis toxicity.

2. Lateral-wall MI, acute. There's a pathologic Q in avl and obvious reciprocal S-T deviation in electrically opposed limb leads. The diagnosis is established beyond question.

3. Right bundle-branch block and anterior MI. The pathologic Q waves establish the diagnosis: Pathologic Q waves are never produced by RBBB per se. There are occasional PVCs arising in the right ventricle. The fifth beat in lead V5 represents normalizing fusion. The narrow beats in V6 may represent normalizing fusion or intermittent bundle-branch block. Prognosis grave! New-onset bundle-branch block with MI implies 50% mortality.

4. Right bundle-branch block and acute anterior MI. The S-T elevation in V2–4 could not possibly be produced by the RBBB: It's characteristic of acute anterior ischemia.

5. Anterior and lateral MI, acute. In the frontal-plane leads there is obvious reciprocal S-T deviation and a lateral Q in avl, all consistent with a lateral MI. There's left anterior hemiblock that appeared acutely with the MI. The precordial leads are a good example of a "Q-equivalent" deflection with no R wave progression at all from V2 to V6. The term "poor R-wave progression" is overused and much abused but as you see it here it's really significant. With left anterior hemiblock it is common to see diminished R-wave progression across the precordial leads, but here there are hardly any R waves at all, even in V5–6.

6. Intermittent WPW, type B. Look at the P-R intervals of the wide beats!

7. LBBB with anterior MI. The pathologic Q waves in the midprecordium and the typical "tombstone" curve of S-T-T in V4–6 are diagnostic. Neither deformity will ever be produced by LBBB.

8. Subnormal sinus node function. Symptoms probably would be vertigo, presyncope, or frank syncope. The wide beats on the left-hand side of the strip are an idioventricular rhythm. There are no visible P waves during this period. The sinus beats on the right-hand side of the strip are conducted with first-degree AV block. If this isn't caused by drugs and if the patient is symptomatic, sick sinus syndrome is present.

9. You can say that this is an abnormal tracing with evidence of myocardial pathology. Period. That's all you can say. You can't say whether the pathology is ischemic or myopathic or degenerative. The symmetrical shape of the inverted T waves makes coronary disease with ischemic pathology more likely than other possibilities, but these are in fact nonspecific T wave deformities and that's all you can call them.

10. Atrial fibrillation with complete AV block and inferior MI. The

possible causes include the AV nodal block commonly seen with inferior MIs or — as in this case — overdose of digoxin.

11. Here and there you see obvious P waves. They appear every three or four beats. If you look at the S-T-T contour of the subsequent beats, you will see that there's a dramatic change in the shape of the T waves. The Q-T interval seems to shorten. Remember that the leopard doesn't change its spots and the T wave doesn't change its shape. Neither does the Q-T interval shorten from beat to beat as it seems to be doing here. When you see either phenomenon, there's a P wave hidden in the T, and that's what's producing the changing morphology. If you measure those odd bumps in the T waves you'll see that they "march out" precisely, yielding an atrial rate of about 152. In other words, PAT is present. Note that each P wave moves closer to the preceding R; this means that the P-R is getting longer, of course. Wenckebach block is present. Put the two diagnoses together and you have PAT with block! Note the dramatic reciprocal S-T deviation: The diagnosis of an acute inferior MI is also obvious.

12. Prolonged Q-T interval. The immediate danger is torsade, and the most common cause is a 1A drug like quinidine. Treatment: discontinue the drug. Treatment of torsade: magnesium sulfate in large doses, IV — also speeding of atrial rate by atrial pacing or atropine.

13. Tough reasoning. There are many narrow QRS complexes that are clearly junctional. There are also P waves. Are these sinus P waves or do they represent retrograde conduction from the junction? Is there any sinus node activity at all? The first beat is clearly junctional: It's followed by a P wave that produces a response. Beat 3 is also junctional, with a P wave half-buried in it. Beat 4 repeats the pattern of beat 1, and so on throughout the strip. In other words, a P wave comes just after one junctional beat and then comes longer after the next junctional beat. After this long R-P there's always an early QRS. Could these P waves be dissociated sinus beats? Of course not — they're always associated with junctional beats! If these were dissociated sinus beats, they'd occur all through the heart cycle, independent of the sinus impulses. This is retrograde Wenckebach from the junction. The first R-P is very short — the P is almost hidden in the QRS. The second R-P is longer, so the AV node has time to recover and conduct back down — reciprocal beating. Full diagnosis: Junctional rhythm with retrograde Wenckebach and reciprocal beating. AV nodal conduction is normal — both retrograde and antegrade. There is no sinus node activity. Sick sinus!

14. The most pronounced form of RVH (Type A). There is also evidence of right atrial enlargement. This type of RVH indicates right-sided pressures close to or equal to arterial pressures. Pulmonic stenosis or

severe pulmonary hypertension secondary to Eisenmenger's patho-physiology will produce this pattern.

15. LBBB with anterior and inferior infarction. LBBB or not, those Q waves are still pathologic and specific!

16. LBBB with unmistakable Pardee (tombstone) configuration of S-T-T in V1–4. LBBB per se will never produce that configuration! Anterior ischemic process, presumably infarction.

17. There's a junctional rhythm with dissociated P waves and three long pauses. The pauses occur when the P wave comes a long time after the QRS. Concealed conduction! When the P wave comes long enough after the junctional beat, it finds the upper nodal tissues out of their refractory period; the sinus impulse penetrates to the site of the junctional pacemaker and resets it. That produces the pause. The lower node is still refractory, so the impulse never reaches the ventricles. Hence the pause. Is complete AV block present? Of course not: The sinus impulse can penetrate to the junctional site to reset it, and the junctional site can reach the ventricles, so there's obviously a track from atria to ventricles. It's just a matter of timing.

18. Wide-beat tachycardia with RBBB configuration and extreme left axis. Fascicular ventricular tachycardia — a distinct entity in terms of mechanism, prognosis, and treatment. These tachycardias are often called "idiopathic ventricular tachycardias," but I think "fascicular" is a better term since it describes the origin and propagation of the impulse.

19. Strip A shows tall, peaked T waves V3–6. Good working rule: When a T wave is more than half the height of an R in a lead that consists primarily of an R, it's significant. Hyperkalemia. Strip B shows sinus rhythm with very wide QRS complexes (about 0.24 seconds). This kind of extreme widening of QRS is strongly suggestive of hyperkalemia, which was in fact present.

20. The wide beats appear after sinus pauses, when the rate slows for one beat. Bradycardia-dependent aberrancy.

21. Wide-beat tachycardia without P waves. Note the alternans in shape and size. This is paroxysmal ventricular tachycardia with electrical alternans, a rare and dangerous arrhythmia usually produced by near-terminal digitalis toxicity.

22. Sinus rhythm with short runs of junctional tachycardia. Note the dramatic increase in S-T elevation with the rapid beating. You're seeing a kind of instant stress test — the more rapid rate is obviously producing increasing ischemia. Slowing the rate will probably be lifesaving; obviously there's a critical lesion in the LAD and this patient is going to need very close attention if not intervention.

23. Atrial fibrillation with very rapid ventricular response. Some of the

R-R intervals are equivalent to a rate of 250 or higher. This always arouses suspicion of preexcitation. Simple test: Give adenosine. If the rate slows, there's no preexcitation; if it speeds, there is. If preexcitation is present, of course, avoid anything that depresses conduction through the AV node.

Warning! When you administer adenosine for possible preexcitation, have a defibrillator ready on standby. During the six seconds of AV nodal blockade the bypass tract can drive the ventricles into ventricular fibrillation. Two such cases have been reported already (see Chap. 11).

24. False alarm! Look at V1 and there's obvious preexcitation. You can also see an obvious delta-R in avl. The Q in avf is simply the "delta-force" of preexcitation, exactly opposite in polarity to the way it appears in avl and V1.

25 | Graduation Exercise

This is a mini-atlas of complex arrhythmias. To analyze them you don't need to learn anything new; you can reach a diagnosis in every case by using the elements you've learned in the text. The trick now is to apply these elements in a logical manner. Each step in the reasoning process is simple, but at the end you'll find you have arrived at diagnosis, prognosis, and treatment in a set of arrhythmias guaranteed to give most of your colleagues a throbbing sense of insecurity.

FIGURE 25-1

This rhythm appeared in the setting of chronic atrial fibrillation. The patient was taking a variety of "heart medicines" but wasn't sure what they were. He presented in the emergency room complaining of "feeling faint as if he was going to pass out." Are impulses from the fibrillating atria reaching the ventricles? If not, what's the rhythm? Is it regular, and if not, is there any pattern? Is AV block present, and if so, where and what kind? How many levels of block do you see?

Answers: First, this is not the helter-skelter ventricular rhythm you expect if the ventricles are responding to fibrillating atria. The rate is slow and the rhythm is almost, but not quite, regular. Impulses from the fibrillating atria are obviously not reaching the ventricles.

Conclusion 1: This is some kind of an "idio" rhythm, presumably arising in the AV junction. It is completely dissociated from the fibrillating atria.

Problem: Junctional rhythms are characteristically completely regular, but this one isn't. If you measure closely you see that the ventricular complexes come progressively closer together, reading from left to right.

In fact the R-R intervals make a nice mathematical progression, measured in seconds: 1.28, 1.20, 1.15, 1.10, 1.05, 1.02, 1.0, 1.0, 0.09. When you see a progressive shortening of R-R intervals, what do you think of? Simple answer: You think of the "typical" form of Wenckebach block! (See Chap. 7 and note item 8 on page 109.)

Conclusion 2: There is a completely dissociated junctional rhythm, and the junctional beats are encountering Wenckebach block in the lower AV node.

Conclusion 3: The R-R intervals at the beginning of the strip equal a rate of 47. You therefore have the criteria for *complete heart block:* complete AV dissociation, a slow ventricular rate, and no capture by an ample number of atrial impulses (about 425 a minute if this is an average atrial fibrillation).

Conclusion 4: There are two levels of AV block:

1. There is complete block between the fibrillating atria and the site of the junctional pacemaker.
2. There is Wenckebach block in the lower node, below the site of the junctional pacemaker.

Final conclusion: The "heart medicine" almost certainly included digitalis, and the treatment simply consisted of withholding the drug. (Note that the digoxin level was 2.2, but the block disappeared completely after the drug was stopped, illustrating once more that you cannot depend on serum levels to diagnose digitalis toxicity. You have to look at the ECG and the patient!)

FIGURE 25-2   The ECG reveals wide QRS complexes *not* preceded by P waves; the rate is normal and the rhythm is slightly irregular. This pattern appeared 12 hours out in the course of an MI; all previous QRS complexes had been narrow.

Differential diagnosis: There are two possibilities:

1. Idioventricular rhythm (benign).

2. Junctional rhythm with new bundle-branch block (bad news: 50% mortality).

The differentiation is critical. You can make it from this strip.

Observation 1: There are obvious atrial complexes. These are diphasic deflections appearing at different intervals after the QRS. Again there are two possibilities: These might be dissociated sinus P waves or retrograde P waves from the ectopic focus.

Answer: If these were dissociated sinus P waves, they would "wander through" the strip with no fixed relation to the QRS. In fact they're always associated with a QRS: If you look closely you see that they come at progressively longer intervals after the QRS. In other words there's a progressive prolongation of the R-P — a *reverse Wenckebach* phenomenon, or as one of my bright students put it, a "Backenwenck." The retrograde P appears as a notch on the first part of the T in beat I, it's farther out into the T in beat II, and it comes at the end of the T in beat III. This pattern repeats itself in the strip so it can't be accidental. These have to be retrograde P waves.

Observation 2: This is really the key. *Beat IV comes early.* The same pattern is repeated in the next four beats; after the longest R-P there's an early QRS. This is reciprocal beating. The retrograde impulse takes so long traveling back up to the atria that the AV tissues have time to recover and the impulse is conducted back down to the ventricles, producing the early beat. The sequence is ventricles-atria-ventricles. The reciprocal beat shows you the pattern of *normal antegrade conduction* just as if it were a normal sinus beat. The QRS of the reciprocal beat is wide, with exactly the same configuration as all the other beats.

Conclusion: The wide beats are the result of bundle-branch block. The pressing clinical problem is solved. This is in fact a junctional rhythm with newly acquired bundle-branch block. The reciprocal beat is the key to the whole diagnosis.

One more refinement: The QRS complexes appear in four-beat cycles. The last beat of each cycle is the reciprocal beat, and of course it's early. Measure the other R-R intervals carefully and you'll find that beats II and III are always closer together than I and II. Again you see that diminishing R-R interval just as in the previous tracing: Wenckebach block! There is antegrade Wenckebach block in the lower node, below the site of the junctional pacemaker.

Final diagnosis: Junctional rhythm with newly acquired bundle-branch block with antegrade and retrograde Wenckebach block and reciprocal beating.

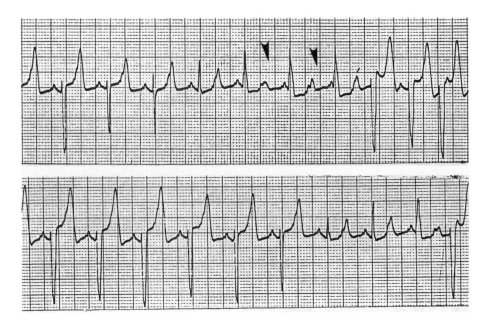

FIGURE 25-3

This patient was sweating, hypotensive, and obviously very sick. He was an elderly member of the Tohono O'Tham tribe (formerly Papagos) of this area and didn't speak much English. He had been taking some kind of medicine he obtained at a free clinic, but nobody knew what it was. The pulse was regular with a rate of 100. The two strips start with a series of beats with a normal P-R (three in the top strip, six on the bottom). Note that the shape of the QRS in these strips changes as you scan from left to right: The QRS becomes progressively narrower and then changes from negative to upright. The beats that consist of an R wave appear at exactly the same rate as the others — they're regular. Now look at the P waves in the series of beats that consist of an R wave. The P-R interval is changing: It seems to be shortening while the ventricular rhythm is regular. A changing P-R interval with a regular ventricular rhythm means dissociation. AV dissociation can take place only when there's an ectopic rhythm. Therefore there must be an idioventricular or idiojunctional rhythm here.

Between the ectopic beats, at the points indicated by arrows, you now see something different — the key to the whole arrhythmia. You see two P waves between each set of ventricular complexes. You now have a chance to measure the atrial rate — it's 250. March your calipers back through the tracing, and you can find this same rapid atrial rate all the way. In the beats that consist of a predominant S wave in the first part of each strip, the alternate P waves appear as a notch on the upslope of the T.

Now you answer two questions:

1. What are the atria doing? They are firing rapidly and regularly at a rate of 215. Diagnosis: paroxysmal atrial tachycardia.
2. Are all the atrial impulses reaching the ventricles? Obviously not. There's 2:1 block in the first part of the tracing and complete dissociation for a period of over two seconds. Diagnosis: AV block.

Put them together: PAT with block!

The peculiar change in QRS morphology is the result of progressive fusion between the sinus impulses and the ectopic rhythm. Since there's fusion, you now know that the ectopic rhythm is an idioventricular rhythm. The normalizing fusion with the narrowing of the QRS tells you that there's really bundle-branch block, even though part of the QRS is hidden in the baseline. (At the right-hand end of each strip, AV conduction resumes with Wenckebach periods.) Stop the digoxin; start the potassium!

FIGURE 25-4   A pacemaker was implanted two years ago for unknown reasons. (They often are!) Now the patient presents with "presyncope" — a slovenly term meaning that sometimes the patient felt some blurring of consciousness "as if he was going to pass out." The ECG tells the whole story. There's a first-degree AV block with bundle-branch block. After three beats there's an abrupt sinus pause. The pause is almost exactly equal to two sinus intervals, so it's true sinoatrial exit block (see Chap. 15). After the sinus pause there's a blocked P wave followed by a paced beat. The same thing happens in the bottom strip — the P wave that comes after a long pause is blocked and the pacemaker discharges.

Here's an odd phenomenon: The atrial complexes that come *late* are blocked; the ones that come earlier are normally conducted. You're looking at bradycardia-dependent refractoriness (Chap. 6). More commonly this phenomenon produces bradycardia-dependent aberrancy, but it can produce bradycardia-dependent block. Since one bundle-branch is blocked, there's only one functioning strand connecting atria and ventricles — a strand consisting of the AV node and the normal bundle branch. The prolonged P-R interval may be the result of delay in the one functioning bundle branch or even in the one functioning fascicle if bifascicular block is present. If bradycardia-dependent refractoriness arises in that one functioning strand, AV conduction will fail when the rate slows, and that's what you're seeing here.

Since this is really intermittent bilateral bundle-branch block, it is in fact a variation of Mobitz-II block, and it has the same dangerous connotations. The patient really needs that pacemaker, but it's not functioning normally. It's firing too slowly (rate about 32) and too late (escape interval about 1.8 seconds). The pacemaker is in urgent need of readjustment or replacement.

FIGURE 25-5   The old bugbear: a wide-beat tachycardia without P waves. This patient had normal narrow QRS complexes on the tracing recorded a few hours previously; this arrhythmia arose in the course of hospitalization for crescendo angina. The ECG presents a simple pattern: It consists entirely

of wide QRS complexes appearing in pairs. There are no atrial complexes anywhere. The beats appear at an interval equal to a rate of 166 (9 squares), then there's a pause that's *less* than double that interval (11 squares).

Answer: Ventricular tachycardia with Wenckebach exit block around the ectopic focus. Why Wenckebach? Remember that with 3:2 Wenckebach block you see two QRS complexes followed by a pause. In any Wenckebach block there's always recovery after the pause; in AV nodal Wenckebach, the P-R interval after the pause *shortens* — it "pulls in" the QRS — so that the pause is less than the sum of the two preceding beats. Same thing with Wenckebach exit block: The pause will always be less than a double interval of the basic rate.

Speculation: When you see exit block during a paroxysmal tachycardia, it's likely that the mechanism is parasystole, rather than reentry. It's easier to conceive of Wenckebach periods around a single ectopic focus than in a reentry loop.

FIGURE 25-6

That was a reasonably straightforward wide-beat tachycardia problem. Now try something challenging. This patient again was severely distressed, with hypotension, sweating, and apprehension. There was a long-standing history of hypertensive heart disease, coronary artery disease, and congestive heart failure, all treated with many drugs by a number of physicians. When the patient presented to the emergency room, he wasn't quite sure which of his numerous medications he'd been taking but he thought they included digoxin.

In this tracing you see narrow and wide QRS complexes, appearing rapidly. The narrow complexes are clearly the result of some kind of supraventricular tachycardia; they appear at a rate of 150. The wide complexes appear at a rate of 125. Those two numbers are the key to the whole arrhythmia. When you see wide QRS complexes, there are two possibilities: ventricular ectopic firing or aberrant conduction. The common type of sustained aberrancy is *rate-dependent aberrancy.* Here the wide QRS complexes appear at a *slower rate* than the narrow ones. You can't invoke aberrancy to explain the wide QRS complexes — they have to be ventricular.

Diagnosis no. 1 is therefore "supraventricular tachycardia interrupted by short runs of ventricular tachycardia." Digitalis toxicity is the presumptive diagnosis. What kind of supraventricular tachycardia? Look at the arrows and you'll see some tiny but well-defined P waves that give you the answer. They appear at exactly the same rate as the narrow complexes. If you look closely you'll see the same tiny P waves in other parts of the strip. The two QRS complexes following the marked P waves are intermediate in shape and size between the wide complexes and the narrow ones. They're *fusion beats,* and that absolutely identifies the wide-beat tachycardia as ventricular.

Now look at the P-R interval of those two beats. It's getting longer. Wenckebach! Look at the T waves of the next five narrow beats and you see small but clear-cut changes as the P moves closer to the preceding T until one is blocked. The P-R is getting longer and the R-P of course is getting shorter. Wenckebach again!

You have now diagnosed the frightening combination of PAT with block and intermittent ventricular tachycardia. This is a potentially lethal combination of digitalis-toxic rhythms. Treatment: Potassium for the PAT with block and diphenylhydantoin for the ventricular tachycardia (it's specific in this setting).

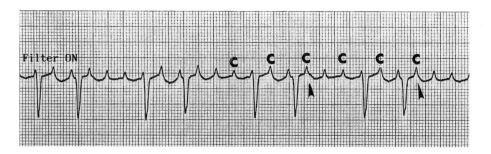

FIGURE 25-7

Atrial flutter with a bigeminal rhythm. Remember that in about one-third of all cases of atrial flutter, the ventricular rhythm is irregular: The ratio of conduction to the ventricles changes from second to second, producing an "irregular irregularity" of the pulse that can't be distinguished from atrial fibrillation at the bedside. Here you have atrial flutter with a "bigeminal," or coupled, rhythm. This coupled rhythm

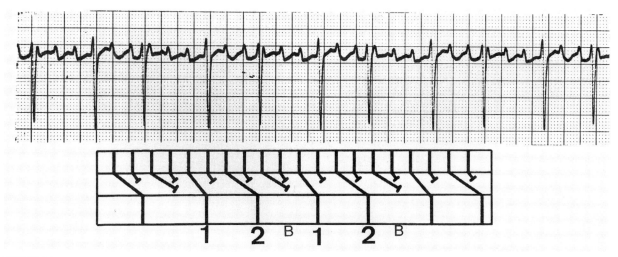

FIGURE 25-8

isn't caused by extra systoles because there is a recurring precise pattern of relationship of flutter waves to QRS throughout. There's a flutter wave about 0.23 seconds ahead of the first QRS of each pair and a flutter wave 0.08 seconds ahead of the second QRS. This precise repetition cannot be accidental. What's going on?

Start with what you know about ordinary 2:1 flutter. Every other flutter wave dies at the AV junction because the AV tissues are refractory — fortunately for the patient. If every flutter wave came through, the heart would race itself to death. The nonconducted flutter waves don't penetrate the AV node at all. Often the flutter impulses that do travel down the AV node will encounter some kind of block. To diagnose the block you must concentrate on the flutter waves that penetrate the AV node — in other words, the alternate flutter waves. You ignore the waves that die at the AV junction.

In Fig. 25-7 the flutter waves that are conducted down the AV node are marked "C." Look at the relation of those waves to the QRS and ignore the other flutter waves because they never really leave the atria. The first "C" is conducted with a P-R of 0.23 seconds. The second is conducted with a P-R of 0.25 seconds. The third is blocked (arrow). The pattern is repeated precisely in the next three "C" beats. You're looking at Wenckebach block of the alternate flutter waves that travel down the AV node. In other words it's an "every-other-beat-Wenckebach."

Again you see two levels of block: one between the atria and the AV node, and the other down in the AV node itself.

Figure 25-8 is a schematic diagram of the same phenomenon. The beats labeled "1" are the first beat of a Wenckebach cycle, the beats labeled "2" are the second, and the blocked beat of course is labeled "B." Note that you ignore the alternate flutter waves that don't penetrate the

AV node. When you're analyzing AV nodal block in the presence of atrial flutter, this is an important concept to keep in mind.

FIGURE 25-9

Figure 25-9 is a really rare bird. It's the only one of its kind I've ever seen, but it illustrates a couple of very basic principles in the diagnosis of wide-beat tachycardia. This woman presented to our clinic describing "dizziness and palpitations."

Most of this tracing is taken up with a totally irregular wide-beat tachycardia without P waves. At first blush you'd think of atrial fibrillation with bundle-branch block. Look again. About two-thirds of the way across the bottom strip you see a normal sinus beat with a narrow QRS.

Next logical question: Why not paroxysmal atrial fibrillation with rate-dependent bundle-branch block? Look at the pause between the fourth and fifth beats in the top strip, and you see a long R-R interval — much longer than the one preceding the narrow sinus beat. If rate-dependent bundle-branch block is causing the wide beats, it should have disappeared after that pause. There's another long pause in the bottom strip, but the wide QRS persists. You have therefore ruled out rate-dependent aberrancy as a cause of the wide QRS complexes. Always be prepared to make this observation when you're analyzing intermittent wide-beat rhythms.

The only other possible cause of a wide QRS is ventricular ectopy. Irregular ventricular tachycardia? It seems unlikely, but look at the beat indicated by the arrow. It's narrow, but the shape of the QRS is definitely different from the two normal beats. The P-R interval is shorter than the P-R of the two normal beats.

Answer — of course: Fusion! You have detected the 100% marker for ventricular ectopy. You have made the very rare but precise diagnosis of "unstable or erratic or variable-rate ventricular tachycardia." This is probably caused by a parasystolic focus with varying degrees of exit block. The principles you used in this rare tracing are the same basic principles you use in analysis of any complex wide-beat tachycardia.

FIGURE 25-10

An intern or a colleague brings you this rhythm strip, muttering about wide beats and some funny kind of ventricular tachycardia. You discover that it was recorded on an elderly patient with severe hypertensive heart disease and an exacerbation of congestive heart failure. The patient had been on many cardiac medications, including antihypertensives, digoxin, and diuretics, in varying combinations at other centers. No previous electrocardiograms are available. Through most of the tracing, wide beats and narrower beats alternate. In the second strip there is a pause punctuated by very wide QRS complexes with a different configuration and a slower rate. Diagnosis? Probable cause? Treatment?

1. There are no P waves anywhere in the tracing, even in the long pause where there should be plenty of time to see them. Presumptive diagnosis: atrial fibrillation.
2. Put your calipers on the *beginning* of the alternating wide and narrow beats and you'll see that the rhythm is absolutely regular.

Conclusion: The wide beats and the narrow beats are coming from the same focus. The narrow beats are too narrow to be ventricular, so they must be junctional.

This is an accelerated junctional rhythm with 2:1 right bundle-branch block. The pattern varies from an "incomplete" to a "complete" RBBB on alternate beats. Accelerated junctional rhythm is the most common sustained digitalis-toxic tachyarrhythmia.

In the pause in the second strip you see a slow rate with very wide

QRS complexes. It looks like typical atrial fibrillation, but if you look closely you'll see that the QRS complexes are quite regular except for the last one, which comes a little early. Clearly this is not the pattern of random conduction from fibrillating atria: This is an idioventricular rhythm. There must be a high degree of AV block since the rate is 68 — plenty of time to allow fibrillary impulses to reach the ventricles if the AV tissues were conducting normally. In fact there's no evidence of conduction from the fibrillating atria to the ventricles anywhere in the tracing. The rhythm is set by two ectopic pacemakers — one junctional and one ventricular. One more time: digitalis toxicity!

FIGURE 25-11   Lead V1, right bundle-branch block. Ventricular ectopic beats forming a "bigeminal" rhythm. Or are they junctional ectopic beats with Ashman aberrancy?

Next day: Still V1, still right bundle-branch block, but the premature beats are narrow!

Analysis: The sinus rate in the first strip is slow. If you count the visible P waves — the little inverted notches ahead of the RBBB beats — it's 40. There might be a P wave hidden in the VPCs, which would give you a sinus rate of 80. In the second strip the sinus rate is much faster — about 106. The right bundle branch is blocked. The VPCs have an LBBB configuration, which means they arise in the right ventricle.

What's happening: In the second strip the rate is much faster. The atrial impulses "get ahead" of the VPCs so that the normal impulse is coming down the right bundle at the same instant that the VPC is activating the left ventricle. Both chambers are discharged at almost the same instant, eradicating the effect of the bundle-branch block for that beat.

It must be normalizing fusion (Chap. 5)! As with any fusion, the P-R of the fused beat is a little shorter than the P-R of the sinus beats. Those premature beats are infallibly identified as ventricular.

Graduation!

26 | How to Take a Board Examination

If you are an intern preparing for boards or a cardiologist preparing for subspecialty boards, or if you want ECG reading privileges at any hospital of any size, you're going to have to take a qualifying examination in electrocardiography. Get used to the idea and prepare for it.

I was the one who launched the idea of the ACC qualifying examination back in the seventies when I served on the continuing education committee of the ACC, and I helped to nurture the project in its early stages as a member of the ECG interpretation committee of the ACC. Under the subsequent able leadership of Drs. Nancy Flowers and Jay Mason, the examination has become an institution. The plan now is to offer it to hospital staffs to qualify physicians for ECG reading privileges, which was what I wanted to do with it in the first place. Dr. H. J. C. Marriott has been offering a similar service to hospitals nationwide for some time, and the enthusiastic reception of his efforts attests a strongly felt need.

Here are some hints on how to approach this kind of examination.

Describe *everything* on the tracing. There will almost always be a number of specific diagnostic deformities and you'll be graded by the number you recognize.

FIGURE 26-1 Diagnosis:

1. Complete AV block, nodal.
2. Inferior myocardial infarction, acute.

That one was easy.

FIGURE 26-2

Here you'll get in trouble unless you look at the rhythm strip on the bottom. The first beat is a normal sinus beat. It's followed by three ventricular beats at a rate of 150. All across the rhythm strip there are occasional sinus beats followed by runs of ventricular ectopic beats and many fusion beats. Now look at the QRST configuration. The whole diagnosis is as follows:

1. Sinus rhythm.
2. Ventricular tachycardia, transient, recurrent.
3. Frequent fusion beats.
4. Anterior myocardial infarction, "hyperacute."

The term "hyperacute" of course refers to the extreme S-T elevation; it's interesting and significant that this elevation is apparent even in the ventricular ectopic impulses. You'll never see S-T elevation like this as part of a VPC per se.

FIGURE 26-3   This will probably bring a question about treatment. This tracing is recorded in an asymptomatic patient. Diagnosis? Pathophysiologic mechanism? Treatment?

1. Sinus rhythm.
2. Ventricular ectopic discharge with
   a. a five-beat run of accelerated idioventricular rhythm with shortening R-R caused by Type 1 exit block.
   b. many fusion beats.
3. Mechanism parasystole. Note varying coupling intervals and interectopic intervals.
4. Treatment: none. (You'll probably be presented with a tempting menu including isoproteronol and pacing. Don't be fooled.)

FIGURE 26-4   This was recorded on a patient complaining of paroxysms of vertigo.

1. Right bundle-branch block.
2. Left anterior fascicular block.
3. Mobitz-II block. (Look at the rhythm strip.)

In this case the Mobitz-II block is a manifestation of *intermittent trifascicular block.* The patient has only one fascicle left, and that's failing now and then.

FIGURE 26-5

1. Atrial flutter.
2. High-degree or complete AV nodal block.
3. Ventricular ectopic beats.

Warning: Whenever you're considering atrial flutter or fibrillation, always assess the degree of AV block — it's a favorite trap.

FIGURE 26-6

1. Junctional rhythm.
2. Inferior MI, acute.
3. Complete sinus arrest.

Here the point is to recognize the acute sinus node suppression, the real cause of the junctional rhythm — a common complication of inferior MIs.

FIGURE 26-7   Left ventricular hypertrophy based on:

1. Increased voltage.
2. "Strain" pattern in S-T-T.
3. Left axis — 30 degrees.
4. Left atrial enlargement.

Don't forget the left atrial enlargement as part of the final diagnosis or you'll lose points.

FIGURE 26-8

1. Atrial fibrillation.
2. Paroxysms of junctional tachycardia (note the absolutely regular tachycardia in the first part of the strip with a rate of 155).
3. Aberrantly conducted junctional ectopic beats (Ashman phenomenon). Note the constant linkage of the wide beats to the preceding narrow beat — this indicates that these are reentrant junctional beats, not random beats from the fibrillating atria.
4. Presumptive diagnosis: digitalis toxicity.

FIGURE 26-9

Runs of paroxysmal atrial tachycardia with RBBB and LBBB aberrancy. Note the obvious P waves at the beginning of each episode and the numerous visible P waves during the runs of LBBB tachycardia. The RBBB tachycardia follows an Ashman pattern with normalization of QRS at the same rate after the three-beat run in the left bottom strip, while the LBBB aberrancy, as usual, is simply rate-dependent. If the examination asks about the type of aberrancy, point out both.

FIGURE 26-10   Favorite booby-trap. Don't call this an inferior MI. It's WPW preexcitation, and the apparent pathologic Q in III and avf is simply the delta-force of preexcitation.

FIGURE 26-11   Examiners love intermittent preexcitation. Don't be misled into calling this a ventricular rhythm — the short P-R and wide QRS are obvious once you're alerted.

FIGURE 26-12   More about aberrancy. You'll probably see a 12-lead ECG like this. The wide complexes appear at a rate of 68. When the rate speeds to 88, the QRS is normal. This is bradycardia-dependent aberrancy, *not* fixed left bundle-branch block.

FIGURE 26-13

Still on the topic of aberrancy:

1. Nonconducted premature atrial beats.
2. Rate-dependent aberrancy.

FIGURE 26-14

Ventricular tachycardia. In any wide-beat tachycardia, be sure to look for evidence of AV dissociation and capture beats with fusion, the two markers for ventricular tachycardia as opposed to aberrancy. The dissociated P waves are obvious, and there's an equally obvious capture beat with fusion right in the middle of the strip.

FIGURE 26-15

They might get tricky on the cardiology boards and hand you something like this. First, note the obvious P waves in the pauses. Second, note the way the apparent Q-T interval shortens. This means that there's a P wave in the T wave moving progressively closer to the preceding QRS as the P-R prolongs. Note also how the R-R interval shortens in each run. Wenckebach!

1. Sinus tachycardia.
2. Type I (Wenckebach) AV block.
3. Inferior MI with hyperacute changes.

I-II-III   aVR-aVL-aVF   V1-V2-V3   V4-V5-V6

Rhythm [II] 10mm/mV

FIGURE 26-16

1. Right ventricular hypertrophy.
2. Right atrial hypertrophy.

Type A RVH; findings consistent with severe pulmonary hypertension.

FIGURE 26-17

You're bound to get one of these. Look for these two elements:

1. A rapid regular atrial rate in the 150–250 range.
2. *Any* degree of AV block: in this case it's 2:1.

PAT with block!

FIGURE 26-18

1. Right bundle-branch block.
2. Left anterior fascicular block — left anterior hemiblock.
3. First degree AV block — trifascicular block.
4. Anterior myocardial infarct.

Don't neglect any of these four items in your diagnosis!

Be sure to review all the infarct patterns and the major arrhythmias in their uncomplicated manifestations. Any examination will consist chiefly of combinations of these elements. Good luck!

Appendixes

Indications for Pacing in the Bradyarrhythmias

The incredibly sophisticated pacemakers available today are a triumph of technology. These instruments can sense the patient's atrial or ventricular complexes and can discharge on demand when the normal rhythm fails for a given period. They can track the patient's own sinus rhythm and can activate the ventricles with a preset P-R interval. They can be programmed to change modes when various rapid rhythms appear, thus protecting the ventricular rate. For those of us who remember the time when there were no such instruments, they are miraculous.

As always, there's another face to the coin. Any time you implant a foreign body in the heart, you have to accept a certain percentage of complications. A permanent pacemaker involves a power pack implanted under the skin and one or, more often, two wires in the heart. Occasional bacteremia and a tendency for blood to clot around foreign bodies must be accepted as a part of the human condition that modern science has not been able to alter. Thus, infection of the pacing apparatus and thrombosis must be anticipated as possible complications.

Most ventricular pacing wires will become permanently attached to the ventricular wall. Like infection around any foreign body, infection of an entrapped pacemaker lead is often resistant to antibiotic therapy and can be controlled only by removing the lead wire. Happily, newer methods of electrode removal by special catheters have reduced the risk inherent in this situation.

In a review that Dr. H. J. C. Marriott and I wrote in the *New England Journal of Medicine* (1985; 312:1428–1432), we noted that the risk of late infection after implantation ranged from 1% to 7% in various reports. A later review by Dr. Seymour Furman, an acknowledged leader in the field of pacemaker technology, documented an 8% risk of infection of lead wires entrapped in the right ventricle in more than 130 patients.

Thrombosis can produce superior vena cava obstruction, massive brachial obstruction, or pulmonary embolization with an overall risk of about 4%.

Socioeconomic implications are serious. Patients wearing permanent pacemakers cannot obtain life insurance or individual health insurance. Many employers are reluctant to hire patients with pacemakers. Many high-frequency energy sources must be avoided (including microwaves).

In other words, the decision to implant a pacemaker must never be made lightly. It's a decision that can alter a patient's whole life.

In the early eighties, I had the privilege of serving as chairman of a committee of distinguished cardiologists who completed a study published under the title of "Indications for Pacing in the Treatment of Bradyarrhythmias" (Phibbs, Friedman, Graboys, Lown, Marriott, Nelson, Preston, *JAMA* 1984;252:1307–1311. The guidelines that follow are derived largely from that report.

In reaching the decision to implant a permanent pacemaker:

1. Rule out drug effect. Repeat that to yourself about a hundred times. Many drugs in common use can depress sinus node function as well as AV and IV conduction. I've tried to emphasize the effects of these drugs in the chapters on heart block and the sick sinus syndrome.

2. Make sure the condition is permanent. Many temporary conditions can affect impulse formation and conduction. Infarcts involving the right coronary artery commonly produce AV nodal block; they can also depress the sinus node. These effects are *always* transient; the patient will *never* need a permanent pacemaker.

3. Rule out extracardiac causes. Electrolyte abnormalities and extreme depression of thyroid function are two obvious examples.

In brief, make sure the condition is stable, permanent, and intrinsic to the heart, then proceed with your decision.

There are only two conditions that warrant pacing in the absence of symptoms:

1. Mobitz-II block localized in the bundle-branch systems.
2. Complete heart-block localized in the bundle-branch system.

Either of these conditions represents a real and present danger to life: the first symptom may be the last. As one example, the rate of catastrophic events with true Mobitz-II block is about 30% per annum. Permanent pacing is indicated whether there are symptoms or not. (That's why we spent so much time in the chapter on heart block talking about these two diagnoses.)

In the conditions listed below, pacing is justified only if the disorder produces symptoms or compromises hemodynamics. "Symptoms" will almost always mean vertigo or syncope; sometimes a sustained slow heart rate will produce chronic fatigue. "Compromised hemodynamics" refers to depressed left ventricular function, usually with some evidence of congestive heart failure.

Complete AV Nodal Block

This is less ominous than complete block localized in the bundle-branch system — that is, it is less likely to lead to syncope or sudden death. Even so, complete AV nodal block will usually require pacing, since the criteria for "complete heart block" include a ventricular rate of 45 or less. Nobody can tolerate a rate that slow forever, and you can be sure there will be symptoms sooner or later. As long as you're quite sure the block is permanent and not caused by extracardiac factors like drugs, pacing is reasonable.

Second-Degree AV Nodal Block

As the student knows, this can take the form of Wenckebach periods or "fixed ratio" block with 2:1 or other conduction. Pacing in this setting is justified only if the block is clearly producing symptoms.

First-Degree AV Nodal Block

First-degree block never justifies pacing.

Atrial Fibrillation with Slow Ventricular Rate

Review the diagnosis of AV block in the setting of atrial fibrillation. If the ventricular rate is slow enough to cause symptoms and if the condition is clearly permanent, pacing is indicated.

Special Categories

Bifascicular Block with Syncope

When bifascicular block is present, conduction from atria to ventricles is reduced to one strand — the one functioning fascicle of the left bundle. If such a patient turns up with recurrent syncope, you might wonder about intermittent failure of that one strand. Careful studies have shown, however, that the risk of this kind of conduction failure is very small. Syncope in the presence of bifascicular block is very rarely the result of a failure of AV conduction. This combination is not per se an indication for pacing.

Trifascicular Block with Syncope

If a patient has right bundle-branch block with hemiblock and if P-R prolongation then appears, it's possible that the delay in AV conduction is in the last remaining fascicle; the term *trifascicular block* is used. Again, careful studies have shown that the risk of progression to Mobitz-II or complete block is small. Pacing is indicated only if actual failure of AV conduction can be demonstrated.

Sick Sinus Syndrome

The sick sinus syndrome, properly defined, is always an indication for pacing. There is no other adequate treatment. When you're considering the diagnosis of "brady-tachy" syndrome, be sure you demonstrate a significant "brady" stage between the episodes of tachyarrhythmia. If you see a normal healthy sinus rhythm in the periods between paroxysms of atrial tachycardia, fibrillation, or flutter, the patient certainly does not need a pacemaker!

Carotid Sinus Syncope

This is a very rare condition. Accidental stimulation of the carotid sinus by movements of the head or neck or by accidental pressure, such as during shaving, will produce abrupt standstill with syncope. In another variation of the syndrome, carotid sinus stimulation causes a drop in blood pressure with syncope. If the "bradycardia" type of carotid sinus syncope is in fact present, pacing is indicated.

Warning: Massaging the carotid sinus will often produce long pauses in the sinus rate. This doesn't mean that carotid sinus syncope is present. It's common to see pauses of 3 seconds or more after carotid massage in perfectly normal people who have never fainted in their lives. In one large series, only 5% of people with pauses of 3 seconds or longer after massage of the carotid sinus actually had clinical carotid sinus syndrome. Drugs that accentuate vagal effect, like digitalis or beta blockers, will produce exaggerated pauses after carotid sinus stimulation.

You can diagnose carotid sinus syncope only when accidental stimulation of the carotid sinus by normal activity causes a pause in heart rhythm or a fall in blood pressure.

Nonindications, Waste Motion, and Booby Traps

In the seventies and eighties there was a wave of enthusiasm for invasive electrophysiologic studies to assess syncope. This led to some spurious indications for pacing, now known to be worthless.

Prolonged H-V Interval
It's possible to measure the interval from the beginning of activation of the His bundle to the beginning of ventricular activation. This interval, also called the H-V interval, is about the last third of the P-R. It is now es-

tablished beyond question that prolongation of the H-V interval per se doesn't mean a thing. Even in the presence of bifascicular block, prolongation of H-V does not indicate increased risk and is not an indication for pacing.

Invasive EP Study of AV Nodal Function

WENCKEBACH PERIODS INDUCED BY ATRIAL PACING. If you place a pacing wire in the right atrium and pace the heart, you'll produce Type I block in almost everybody. In some the block will appear at rates as low as 75–80, while in others it won't appear until the rate is over 150. Wenckebach block induced by artificial pacing is a meaningless finding. It has no correlation with intrinsic block in the AV node. The rate at which Wenckebach periods appear — the so-called Wenckebach number — has no significance in terms of AV nodal function in real life.

INVASIVE EP MEASUREMENT OF FUNCTIONAL AND EFFECTIVE AV NODAL REFRACTORY PERIODS. If the P-R interval on the surface ECG is normal and remains normal throughout any and every variation of rate, there's nothing wrong with the AV node. That's all you need to know about the AV node. Invasive measurements of AV nodal refractory periods serve no useful purpose and have no predictive or prognostic value.

"CHRONOTROPIC INCOMPETENCE." This is a mysterious entity that was used to justify many pacemaker implantations a few years back. The idea was that the sinus node couldn't speed up on demand the way it was supposed to so that a patient might feel weak or dizzy with exertion because the heart rate was too slow to meet the increased demand. There never was any evidence for the existence of such a syndrome and the notion has been discarded, but you may still encounter patients wearing pacemakers for treatment of this mythical disorder.

INVASIVE ELECTROPHYSIOLOGIC MEASUREMENT OF SINUS NODE FUNCTION. Several methods were devised to measure sinus node function in questionable cases of sick sinus syndrome. These included measurement of the pause after rapid pacing and estimation of conduction time from sinus node to atria. Neither of these measurements were very reliable, and the invention of event recorders has made them obsolete. To diagnose sick sinus syndrome, you record sinus node slowing during symptoms by means of Holter recording or with the event recorder — that's the gold standard. Invasive measurements are useless and may be misleading.

How to Determine Axis

You've probably learned some of the "shorthand" ways of determining frontal-plane axis. Thus the axis will be at right angles to the lead that's isoelectric — in other words, the lead that has a total amplitude sum of zero. That's correct, but limited. Sometimes there's no lead like that. You may have learned to derive axis from lead I and avf, but when you

FIGURE A-1
The triaxial system with all leads reduced to a common center.

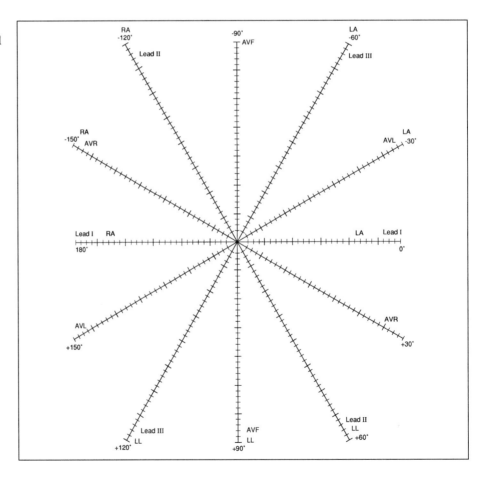

FIGURE A-2
This is "normal" axis. Many texts state that a "normal" axis lies between 0° and +90°. This is dangerously misleading. You have to correct for age and body habitus before you decide whether an axis is normal.

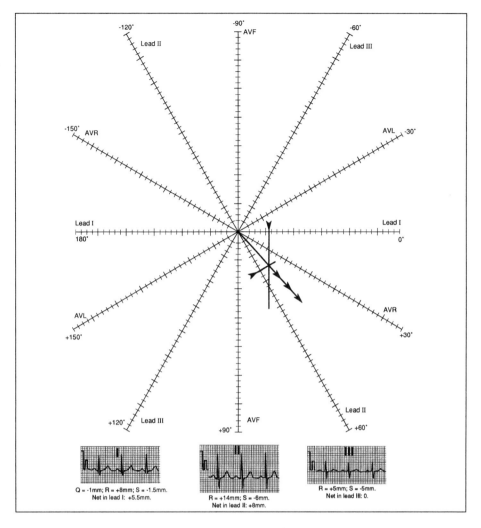

Q = -1mm; R = +8mm; S = -1.5mm.
Net in lead I: +5.5mm.

R = +14mm; S = -6mm.
Net in lead II: +8mm.

R = +5mm; S = -5mm.
Net in lead III: 0.

combine a standard lead with an augmented limb lead it's like combining centimeters and inches — the leads represent different electric magnitudes and you'll be off by exactly ten degrees. Sometimes that can be a significant error.

Here's the right way to go about it. Start with the triaxial system with all leads reduced to a common center (Fig. A-1). Look at the ECG illustrated in the upper left corner of Fig. A-2 and go through the drill outlined there. You simply determine the algebraic sum of deflections in any two leads and mark off that amount on the appropriate lead. Remember that the left arm is plus in lead I and the left leg is plus in leads II and III. Now drop perpendiculars from the points you've measured to

FIGURE A-3
Left axis deviation. The plus value in lead I is the same as the minus value in lead III. You're bisecting the angle between lead I (0) and lead III (−60), just the way you did in high school geometry. Lead II is exactly zero. The perpendicular from lead II points out along the −30 line. This is the other way you can diagnose an axis of −30. Remember, the axis will always be at right angles to the lead that equals zero, just the way it is here. If lead II is zero, the axis will be ±30°. If lead I is zero, the axis will be ±90°. The other leads will tell you at once whether the value is plus or minus either way.

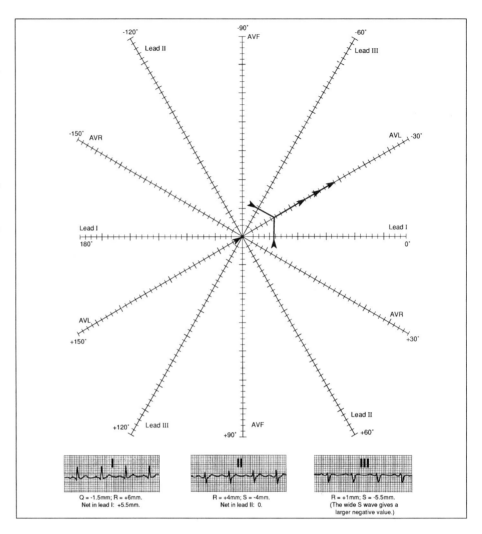

the point of intersection and draw an arrow from the center to that point. That's the mean axis. It's really the simple vector analysis you learned in high school to determine the mean vector of two forces.

Now consider left axis deviation as in Fig. A-3. Leads I and III give exactly the same value except that lead I is plus and lead III is minus. Plot the values, drop the perpendiculars, and you'll find you've bisected the angle between 0 and 60 degrees: 30 degrees. Next important point: The value of lead II is exactly zero. Draw a perpendicular from the zero point on lead II and you're pointing right out at minus 30 degrees. This time the isoelectric lead trick worked.

Extreme left axis is illustrated in Fig. A-4. Rule: When the negative

FIGURE A-4
Extreme left axis deviation. The negative value in III is greater than the plus value in I. Lead II is negative. By looking at the graph you'll see at once that both these findings put the axis leftward of −30° — up in the range of −45° or higher. (Remember, "higher" means "more leftward.")

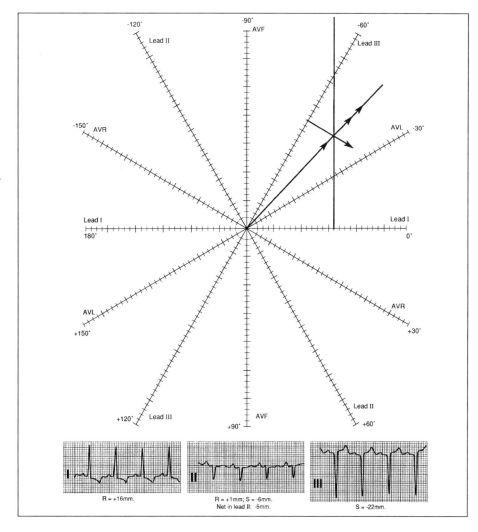

value of III is greater than the plus value of I, the axis will lie leftward of minus 30 degrees. Lead II will always be negative in this setting. Try various values on the triaxial sheet and you'll see how it works.

Right axis deviation (Fig. A-5): some simple rules:

1. If lead I is exactly zero, the axis must point straight up or straight down — plus or minus 90 degrees.
2. If II and III are plus, the axis must point down, at plus 90 degrees.
3. If lead I is negative and II and III are plus, the axis must lie to the right of 90 degrees — about plus 12 degrees in the example here.

FIGURE A-5
Right axis deviation. Whenever lead I is minus and II and III are plus, the way they are here, the axis has to be somewhere to the right of +90°. Try moving the lead I value farther to the minus side, and you'll see values of +110, +120, and so on. Simple concept.

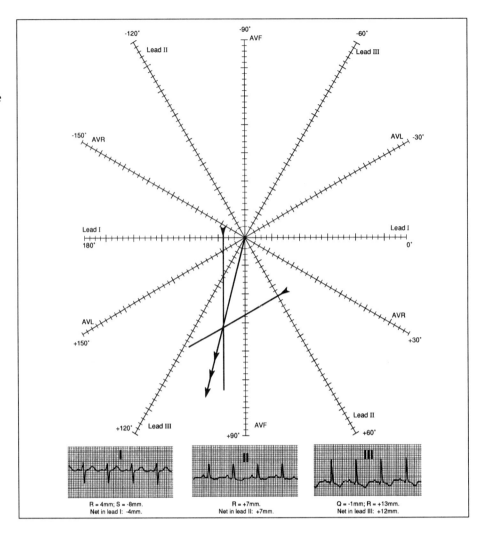

R = 4mm; S = -8mm.
Net in lead I: -4mm.

R = +7mm.
Net in lead II: +7mm.

Q = -1mm; R = +13mm.
Net in lead III: +12mm.

4. If lead II is exactly zero, lead I is negative, and lead III is plus, the axis will be at right angles to lead II, or plus 150 degrees.

And so on. Play around with some values on a sheet with the triaxial lead system and you'll be able to derive axis by simple inspection very accurately.

Index

Aberrancy, 28, 30–31, 61–69,
134
  Ashman. *See* Ashman aberrancy
  bradycardia-dependent. *See*
    Bradycardia-dependent aber-
    rancy
  diagnosing, 29, 129–130
  Phase 4. *See* Bradycardia-
    dependent aberrancy
  prolongation of refractory period,
    61
  random, non-rate-dependent, 61,
    68–69
  rate-dependent, 20, 21, 61, 65, 342,
    357
  transient, 19
  ventricular, 19
Aberrant conduction, 129–130
Ablation, 85
Abrupt pause, 110, 111, 112
ACC Competency Test, 4, 348
Accelerated idiorhythms, 12–14, 71,
    74, 83, 130, 131, 152, 159, 187
Accelerated junctional rhythms, 74,
    83, 187, 345
Adenosine, 30, 33, 36, 135, 144, 170
  defibrillator standby with, 171, 334
AIDS, 291
Akhtar, 27
Amiodarone, 180, 204
Angina pectoris, 267
Anterior fascicular block, 53, 352
Antidepressants, 309

Arrhythmias, 23
  digitalis-toxic, 42, 206–217, 306
  fatal, 169, 191–197
  hypoxic, 42
  interference-dissociation, 100
  of "irregular irregularity," 125,
    212, 342
  preexitation and, 167
  sinus, 2–3, 68
  ventricular fibrillation, 191, 192,
    305
  ventricular standstill, 191, 196, 305
Ashman aberrancy, 61, 62–65, 75, 76,
    84, 112–113, 114, 128, 354
  delayed Ashman reset, 64–65, 66,
    76, 77, 84
Asystole, Mobitz-II block and, 95
Atrial beats, premature, 75, 76, 78,
    84, 111–114
Atrial ectopic beats, 5
Atrial enlargement, 279–280
Atrial fibrillation, 42, 63–64,
    125–137, 215, 322, 331, 354
  AV block in the presence of,
    132–133
  bypass tracts with, 167–175
  character of the fibrillary waves,
    125–128
  coarse. *See* Flutter-fibrillation
  with complete AV block, 133
  diagnosis of, 125, 329, 333
  digitalis toxicity and, 214–217
  with ectopic beats, 128–130

Atrial fibrillation—continued
  pacing and, 365
  and paroxysmal tachycardia,
    133–135
  with rate-dependent bundle-
    branch block, 135–136
  with slow ventricular rate, 132, 365
  treatment of, 169, 214
  ventricular rhythm becomes regu-
    lar during, 130–132
Atrial flutter, 138–150, 153, 156, 157,
    159, 212
  diagnosis of, 138, 144–147, 212,
    342, 352
  exercise-induced, 149–150
  1:1 flutter, avoiding, 148–150
  identifying flutter waves, 141–143
  treatment of, 148, 213, 307
  Wenckebach block in presence of,
    147–148
Atrial kick, 74, 83
Atrial pacing, 84
Atrial premature beats. See Ectopic
    beats
Atrial tachycardia, multifocal, 78, 84
Atrio-ventricular dissociation. See
    AV dissociation
Atropine, 83–84, 194, 208, 332
Automatic-demand "idio"pacemak-
    ers, 11–12
  accelerated, 12–14
Automatic ectopic beating, 10–16
  accelerated idiorhythms, 12–14
  automatic-demand, 11–12
  automatic-parasystolic, 14–16
  automatic tachycardias, 14
  distinguishing between, 10–16
Automatic ectopic focus, 11
Automatic junctional tachycardia
    (nonparoxysmal), 32, 37–39
Automatic-parasystolic firing, 14–16
AV block, 86–109
  with atrial fibrillation, 132, 133
  with bundle-branch block, 87, 88,
    93–94, 97, 118, 121, 152, 159, 160
  classifying, 87–90

complete. See Complete heart
    block
  concealed His bundle beats,
    115–117
  diagnosis of complex forms of,
    110–124
  digitalis-induced, 208, 214–215
  first-degree, 87, 89, 90, 365
  "fixed ratio," 87, 92–94
  high-degree, 110
  interference-dissociation and,
    215
  intra-Hisian, 122–123
  Langendorf-Pick principle,
    117–122
  localizing, 87
  Mobitz-II. See Mobitz-II block
  pseudoblock, 110–117, 124, 203
  P wave shortage, 123–124
  second-degree, 87, 90–98, 365
  sites of, 86–87
  third-degree, 87
  Type II. See Mobitz-II block
  Type I. See Wenckebach block
  Wenckebach. See Wenckebach
    block
AV conduction, 54–55
AV dissociation, 17, 21–23, 26, 39,
    98–104, 123, 133, 146, 156, 160,
    215, 336
  two types of, 99–100
AV nodal reciprocating tachycardia
    (AVPET), 32, 35–37, 37
  treatment, 36–37
AV nodal reentrant tachycardia
    (AVNRT), 31–35, 36, 37
  diagnosis of, 79, 85
  mechanism of, 32, 34
  treatment, 33
AV node, cells in, 86
Axis, 78, 84, 176
  age and habitus and, 278
  calculating, 56, 278, 368–372
  left deviation, 57, 372, 373
  "normal," 278, 369
  right deviation, 371, 372

Bazett formula, 196–197
Beryllium, 291
Beta-blocking drugs, 169, 180, 194, 204
Bifascicular block, 43, 51–58, 112
    pacing and, 365–366
Bigeminal rhythm, 147–148, 201, 342, 346
Bipolar system, 294–295
Board examination, how to take, 348–359
Bradyarrhythmias, indications for pacing in, 363–367
Bradycardia-dependent aberrancy, 61, 65–67, 68, 190
    diagnosis of, 80, 85, 327, 329, 333, 340, 356
Bradycardia-tachycardia syndrome, 201–204, 205
    diagnosis of, 203
Breathing cycle, 2–3
Brugada, 27
Bundle-branch block, 17, 18–21, 337
    AV block with, 87, 88, 93–94, 97, 118, 121, 152, 159, 160
    complete, 45, 46
    diagnosing myocardial infarction in the presence of, 254–266
    incomplete, 43, 45–47, 48, 49
    intermittent, 43, 47–48, 49, 50, 93
    normal conduction, 20, 21
    quinidine and, 309
    rate-dependent, 17, 19–21, 76, 77, 84, 118, 135–136, 158, 160
    See also Left bundle-branch block (LBBB); Right bundle-branch block (RBBB)
Bundle-branch Wenckebach, 183, 189–190
Bypass tracts, 35, 36
    and "artificial" QRS deformity, 171
    with atrial fibrillation, 167–175
    James fiber, 165
    Kent bundle, 162, 164
    See also Preexcitation

Calcium, 303
Calcium-blocking drugs, 169, 204
Capture beats, 17, 25–29, 121
Cardiac arrest, 196
Cardiac sarcoid, 52
Cardiovascular Boards, 4
Carotid sinus massage, 33, 135, 170
Carotid sinus pressure, 74, 121, 138
Carotid sinus stimulation, 74, 83, 84, 89, 144, 149–150, 170
Carotid sinus syncope, pacing and, 366
Catastrophic asystole, 95
"Cavity" of the heart, negatively charged, 293
"Cavity" potential, 235
Cell activation phase, between beats, 67
Cells
    AV node, 86
    sinus node, 186
Chagas's cardiomyopathy, 296
Chamber enlargement, 278–290
    dilatation and hypertrophy and, 278–279
    ECG and, 279–280, 281–284, 284–287
    left ventricular hypertrophy, 281–284
    "normal" axis and, 278
    right ventricular hypertrophy, 284–287
Childhood tachycardia, 32, 39, 40, 41
Chronic lung disease, with hypoxemia, 78, 84
Chronic obstructive lung disease, 286–287
Clonidine, 124, 204
Cocaine, 291
Cocaine addicts, 218
Complete AV nodal block. See Complete heart block

Complete heart block, 98–109, 119,
123, 133, 146, 151, 152, 155, 159,
160
and concealed conduction, 186
diagnosis of, 158, 161, 322, 331,
336, 349
high-degree, 352
pacing with, 365
Complete sinus arrest, 352
Concealed conduction, 132, 327,
333
ECG recognition of, 183–186
Concealed His bundle beats
Conduction
aberrant, 129–130
concealed, 132, 183–186, 327, 333
irregular, 152, 159
measuring, 183
normal antegrade, 337
retrograde, 72, 82, 83, 85, 115
speed of, 6, 9
supernormal, 183, 188–190
WPW, 162–164, 165
Congenital abnormality, 193
Congestive heart failure, 169, 198
Coronary artery disease, 291
Coronary node, 1
"Cove-plane" configuration, 221
Crescendo angina, 340
Cumming, G., 282

Defibrillator, 171, 194
Delta waves, 162–163, 170, 171
Devereaux, M., 283
Diagnosis, exercises in, 335–359
Digitalis, 29, 36, 114, 149, 169, 170,
204
defined uses of, 206
measuring levels of, 209–210
"Digitalis effect," 307
Digitalis toxicity, 38, 42, 118, 129,
133, 152, 306–307
arrhythmias, 42, 206–216, 306
and atrial fibrillation, 214–217
diagnosis of, 159, 206–209, 336,
346, 354

diagnostic algorithm for, 217
PAT with block, 210–213
Digoxin, 313
Dilatation, 278–279
Diphenylhydantoin, 217, 342
Disopyramide, 309
Dissociated P waves, 74, 83
Dissociation, 17, 21–23, 26, 39
interference, 72, 83
intermittent, 158, 161
See also AV dissociation
Diving reflex, 29, 33
Dressler beats, 23
Drug effect, 68, 108
Drugs, 306–307
antiarrhythmic, 204
antidepressant, 309
beta-blocking, 169, 180, 194, 204
calcium-blocking, 169, 204
depressant, 307
that depress sinus node function,
204
digitalis, 306–307
opium derivatives, 204
psychotropic, 204
suppressant, 36, 114, 205
tricyclic, 108, 309
Dual AV nodal pathways, 31, 33
Dyspnea, incapacitating, 198

ECG, limitations of, 291
ECG competency test, 4
ECG privileges examination, 4
Ectopic atrial rhythms, 2
Ectopic atrial tachycardia of childhood, 32, 39, 40, 41, 83, 85
treatment of, 85
Ectopic beats, 4–16
accelerated automatic-demand,
12–14
accelerated idiorhythms, 15
atrial, 5, 9–10, 75, 76, 78, 84,
111–114, 128
atrial, blocked, 111, 112
atrial fibrillation with, 128–130
automatic, 10–16

automatic-demand, 11–12, 15
automatic-parasystolic, 14–16
automatic tachycardia, 16
causal connection with sinus beat, 9
determining source of, 4–8
digitalis and, 208
digitalis toxicity, 216
fascicular, 178–179
junctional, 6–7, 9–10, 128
mechanisms of, 9–16
reentrant, 15, 129
reentrant ventricular, 9–10
ventricular, 7–8, 9–10
width of, 176–177
Ectopic firing, 39
wandering pacemaker distinguished from, 1
Ectopic rhythms, 21–22
sustained, 4–16
Electric shock, 194
Electrive cardioversion, principle of, 195
Electrolyte intoxication, 68
Electrolytes, 303–306
Electrophysiologic (EP) studies, 177, 180
invasive, 366–367
Emphysema, 53, 287
Encainide, 169
Epicardium, 273
Escape beating, 201, 203
Escape interval, 11, 13
Estes, E. H., 282
Event recorder, 205
Examinations, how to take, 348–359
Exercise, 149–150, 199
Exit block, 186–188, 199
sinoatrial, 187, 188
Wenckebach type, 187–189, 341

FAB fragments, 217
Fascicles, 177
Fascicular beats, anterior, 177
Fascicular blocks, 43, 51–58, 352

defined, 51–52
pacing and, 365–366
Fascicular tachycardia, 8, 176–182, 327, 333
anterior, 179, 182
Fibrillary waves, 126, 151, 159
appearance inside the atria, 137
"Fixed ratio" block, 87, 92–94
Flecainide, 169
Flowers, Nancy, 348
Flutter, 63, 64
Flutter-fibrillation, 126, 127, 128, 151, 155, 159
Flutter waves, 126, 138–140
characteristics of, 141–143, 213
Wenckebach block of alternate, 343
Full compensatory pause, 8
Fusion, 17
Fusion beats, 23, 24, 25, 26, 84, 133–134, 342, 350

Goldberger, 229
Gorlin, R., 223

Heart cycle, vulnerable zone of, 194–195
Hemiblocks, 43, 51–58, 78, 84
defined, 53
High-degree block, 110
His bundle, 122–123
His bundle beats, 115–117
Holter monitor, 272
"Hunk disease," 291
Hurst, W., 291
Hypercalcemia, 303
Hyperkalemia, 204, 303, 327, 328, 333
Hyperpotassemia, 304
Hypertrophy, 222, 278–279
of ventricular musculature, 281–284
Hypocalcemia, 303, 304
Hypokalemia, 306
Hypothermia, 311–312

Hypothyroidism, 204
Hypoxemia, 78, 84
Hypoxic arrhythmia, 42

Idiojunctional rhythm, 12–14
  accelerated, 74, 83, 187, 345
Idiopathic ventricular tachycardia,
  180–181, 327, 333
Idiorhythms, 10, 12, 335
  accelerated, 12–14
  sustained accelerated, 14
Idioventricular rhythm, 12–14,
  339
  accelerated, 71, 83, 130, 131, 152,
  159
Image cancellation, 218
Inappropriate sinus bradycardia,
  198–199
Infarct pattern, 218, 220, 224
Instrinsicoid deflection, 282
Interference-dissociation, 100, 101,
  102, 103, 104
  and AV block, 215
Intermittent aberrancy, 61, 67–69
Intermittent bilateral bundle-branch
  block, 93, 95
Intermittent bundle-branch block,
  43, 47–48, 49, 50
Intermittent interference-dissociation, 101
Intermittent trifascicular block, 352
Internal Medicine Boards, 4
Intra-Hisian block, 122–123
Intravenous diphenylhydantoin,
  217
Intravenous magnesium, 42, 193
Intravenous potassium, 210
Intraventricular conduction, 43–60
  fascicular blocks, 43, 51–58
  "incomplete," 43, 45–47, 48, 49
  intermittent bundle-branch block,
  43, 47–48, 49, 50
  nonspecific delay, 43, 58–59
  normalizing fusion, 48–51
Invasive EP study of AV nodal function, 366–367

Ischemia, 68, 221, 269, 271
  acute, 218, 219, 257, 268, 357, 368
  acute, anterior, 265
  See also Transient myocardial ischemia (TMI)
Ischemic cardiomyopathy, 291
Isoproteronol, 194

James fiber bypass, 165
Josephson, M., 27
Junctional escape beating, 201
Junctional rhythms, 80, 85, 332, 337,
  352
  accelerated, 72, 83, 187, 345
  digitalis-toxic, 209
  pause in, 184, 185
Junctional tachycardia, 6–7, 29, 117,
  133, 134, 354
  with bundle-branch block, 17
  compared to ventricular, 7

Kent bundle bypass, 162, 164

Langendorf-Pick principle, 117–
  122
Lang-Jervil-Niellsen syndrome,
  193
Left anterior hemiblock, 57, 359
Left bundle-branch block (LBBB),
  18, 20, 51
  diagnosis of, 79, 81, 84, 85, 320,
  326, 331, 333
  myocardial infarction in presence
  of, 256–258, 259–266
  progression from incomplete to
  complete, 189
Left ventricular hypertrophy (LVH),
  281–284, 353
Lidocaine, 29, 77, 112, 180
Lie, 27
Lown, Bernard, 114, 194
Lown-Ganong-Levine (LGL) preexitation, 164–166, 167
Low serum potassium, 195, 210
Lupus erythematosus, 291
Lyons, T. P., 282

Magnesium sulfate, 332
Mahaim fiber preexitation, 166
Marriott, H. J. C., 27, 114, 348, 363
Mason, Jay, 348
Mitral disease, 279
Mobitz-II block, 87, 94–98, 111–112,
    114, 116, 122, 187
  atypical, 117–122, 154, 157, 160
  diagnosis of, 152, 159
  digitalis toxicity and, 208
  within the His bundle, 122
  pause in, 187
  pseudo-, 115–117, 124
Morphine, 204
Multifocal atrial tachycardia (MAT),
    2, 5, 6, 32, 40–42
Myocardial infarction, 43, 113, 204,
    218–253
  acute, 129, 224, 349, 352
  anterior, 225, 228, 255, 256, 315,
    316, 317, 320, 331, 350, 359
  detecting an infarct and localizing
    it anatomically, 225–228
  diagnosis of, 46, 48, 49, 171, 218,
    221, 223, 229–230
  ECG and, 229–230, 234–253
  hyperacute, 350, 357
  infarct pattern, 218, 220, 224
  inferior, 108, 224, 237, 238, 264,
    322, 331, 349, 352, 357
  lateral, 317, 331
  lateral-wall, 314, 331
  pathologic Q waves, 221, 222, 225,
    233, 256, 260
  posterior, 225–228, 239
  in presence of LBBB, 256–258,
    259–266
  in presence of RBBB, 254–257
  Q wave equivalent deformities,
    230–233, 234
  reciprocal pattern, 218, 220,
    223–224, 227
  right ventricular, 228
Myocardial ischemia, 195. *See also*
    Transient myocardial ischemia
    (TMI)

Myocardial pathology, evidence of,
    331
Myocardium, 273

Narrow beats, 64–65
"Narrow VPC," 176–177
Nitroglycerine, 268
Non-rate-dependent aberrancy, 61,
    67–69
Nonspecific intraventricular con-
    duction delay, 43, 58–59
"Nonspecific" myocardial pathol-
    ogy, 291–302
  ECG diagnosis, 292–296
Normalizing fusion, 48–51, 347
  mechanism of, 50

One-way block, 9–10
"Osborne wave," 311–312

Pacemakers ectopic, 119, 154, 157,
    160, 199, 200, 363
  automatic-demand, 11–14
  "demand" ectopic, 204
  reserve, 10
Pacing artificial, 108, 194, 205
  with atrial fibrillation, 365
  with bifascicular block and syn-
    cope, 365
  in bradyarrhythmias, 363–367
  with carotid sinus syncope, 366
  with complete AV nodal block,
    365
  with first- and second-degree AV
    nodal block, 365
  indications, 364
  nonindications, 366–367
  presyncope and, 339–340
  risk of infection with, 363
  with sick sinus syndrome, 366
  with trifascicular block and syn-
    cope, 365
Parasystole, 14–15, 351
Parasystolic focus, 14–16

Parasystolic rhythms, 16
Paroxysmal atrial tachycardia, 77,
    84, 354
  with block, 42
Paroxysmal junctional tachycardia,
    208
Paroxysmal supraventricular tachy-
    cardia, 31, 63, 79, 85, 167, 168,
    169, 329, 333
Paroxysmal tachycardia, 9–10, 36,
    208, 216, 341
  atrial fibrillation and, 133–135
Paroxysmal ventricular tachycardia,
    177
Pathologic state, 267
PAT with block, 210–213, 217, 323,
    332, 339, 344, 358
Pericarditis, 273–277
  acute, 274
Peri-infarction block, 59
Phase 4 aberrancy. *See* Bradycardia-
    dependent aberrancy
Phase-4 depolarization, 67
Phenothiazines, 309
Phenylephrine, 29
"P-mitrale," 279
Polyarteritis nodosa, 291
Postectopic pause, 85
Posterior fascicular block, 54
Posterior hemiblock, 53, 54
Potassium, 195, 210, 303, 342
  high levels of, 108
"P-pulmonale," 279
Preexcitation, 7, 162–175, 330,
    334
  and arrhythmias, 167
  importance of, 167, 168, 169
  intermittent, 174, 356
  WPW, 162–164, 165, 355
  See also Bypass tracts
Preexcitation tachycardia. *See* AV
    nodal reciprocating tachycardia
    (AVPET)
Premature beats. *See* Ectopic beats
Presyncope, 198, 339–340
Prinzmetal, M., 233

Procaine amide, 29, 36, 148, 169, 180,
    204, 309
Prolonged H-V interval, 366–367
Prolonged Q-T interval, 195
Propafenone, 204
Proudfit, W., 282
Pseudoblock, 110–115, 124, 203
Psychotropic drugs, 204
Pulmonary embolus, 278, 310–311
Pulmonary hypertension, 53, 279
Pulmonic stenosis, 286
Purkinje fibers, 9
P wave shortage, 123–124

"QS" complex, 236
Q-Tc, 196–197
Q-T interval
  measurement of, 196–197
  tables, 197
Quinidine, 29, 36, 114, 148, 169, 180,
    193, 204, 303, 307–309, 332
Q waves, 43–44, 229
  equivalent deformities, 230–233,
    234
  genesis of, 44, 46
  misreading, 44
  normal septal, 43–45
  pathologic, 43, 44, 221, 222, 225,
    233, 256, 260
  transmural and subendocardial,
    233
  width of, 43–44

Reciprocal pattern, 218, 220,
    223–224, 227
Reciprocating, 31
Reentrant ectopic beats, 129
Reentrant ventricular ectopic beats,
    9–10, 208
Reentry, 9–10, 85, 152, 159
Refractory period
  heart rate and, 62–63
  prolongation of, 61
Reicheck, R., 283
Reserve pacemakers, 10
Respiratory variations, 3

Retching, 12
Retrograde conduction, 72, 82, 83,
  85, 115
Right atrial hypertrophy, 358
Right bundle-branch block (RBBB),
  19, 112, 119, 133, 134, 164, 296
  diagnosis of, 74, 79, 81, 83, 84, 85,
    320, 325, 326, 331, 352, 354, 359
  myocardial infarction in presence
    of, 254–257
  T waves and, 254, 257
Right ventricular hypertrophy
  (RVH), 53, 284–287, 324, 332, 358
Romano-Ward syndrome, 193
Romhilt, D.W., 282
R-on-T phenomenon, 194–196

Sarcoidosis, 291
Scar tissue, 291
Schmock, Carl, 286
Scleroderma, 291
Self-assessments, 71–85, 151–161,
  313–334
Sick sinus syndrome, 2, 198–205,
  206, 323, 332
  diagnosis of, 198–204, 205
  mystery of, 204–205
  pacing and, 366
  treatment of, 205
Silent myocardial ischemia, 272
Sinoatrial block, 200
Sinoatrial node, cells of, 198
Sinus arrhythmia, 2–3, 68
Sinus beat, causal connection with
  ectopic beat, 9
Sinus bradycardia, 124
  inappropriate, 198–199
Sinus node, 186
Sinus node function, 2
  subnormal, 320, 331
Sinus node reentrant tachycardia,
  32, 39–40, 41
Sinus pause, 12, 199
Sinus pauses
  random, 200
Sinus rhythm, 1–3, 329, 333, 350, 351

interrupted, 76
two benign variations, 1–3
Slow/fast track, 32, 34
Sokolow, M., 282
Sotalol, 180, 204
Spodick, David, 274, 277
Spontaneous angina, 269
Standstill. See Ventricular standstill
ST segments
  horizontal or downsloping de-
    pression of, 269, 270, 271
  "junction" depression of, 269
  and Pardee "cove-plane" curve,
    221
  "Tombstone" configuration, 221,
    254, 255, 256, 257, 263
Supernormal conduction, 183,
  188–190
Suppressant drugs, 36, 114, 205
Supraventricular tachycardias,
  31–42, 79, 342
  automatic junctional, 32, 37–39
  AV nodal reciprocating, 32, 35–37
  AV nodal reentrant, 31–35
  with delayed Ashman reset, 76,
    77, 84
  ectopic atrial, 32, 39, 40, 41
  multifocal atrial, 32, 40–42
  paroxysmal atrial with block, 42,
    79, 85
  sinus node reentrant, 32, 39–40, 41
  treatment, 29, 30
  types of, 31
Sustained ectopic rhythms, 10
Syncope, 198, 205, 365–366

Thrombolysis, 224
Thrombolytic therapy, 71
Thrombosis, 363–364
Thrombus, 218, 219
Torsade, 192–194, 196, 309, 332
  treatment of, 193–194
Transient myocardial ischemia (TMI)
  evidence of, 267, 272
  symptoms of, 267
"Treppe" or "steps," 310

Tricyclic drugs, 108
 antidepressants, 309
Trifascicular block, 43, 51–58, 352, 359
 pacing and, 365–366
Two-track AV nodal reentry tachycardia. *See* AV nodal reentrant
 tachycardia (AVNRT)
Type I block. *See* Wenckebach block
Type II block. *See* Mobitz-II block

Unipolar limb leads, 229

Vagal stimulation, 29, 33, 36, 170,
 204
 in diagnosis of flutter, 144–147
Vagus nerve, overstimulation of,
 206–207
Valsalva maneuver, 29, 33
Ventricular ectopic beats, 7–8, 154,
 160
 compared to junctional, 7
 diagnosing, 64
 reentrant, 9–10
Ventricular ectopy, 344, 346, 351, 352
Ventricular fibrillation, 191, 192, 305
 coarse, 192
 "fine," 191
Ventricular flutter, 192
Ventricular fusion, 48, 50
Ventricular rhythm
 regular, during atrial fibrillation,
 130–132
 irregular, 125, 139, 146
Ventricular standstill, 191, 196, 305
Ventricular tachycardia, 8, 17, 26, 29,
 177, 178
 diagnosis of, 72, 73, 74, 75, 82, 83,
 84, 341, 350, 357
 digitalis-toxic, 209
 idiopathic, 180–181, 327, 333

Verapamil, 29, 169, 170, 178
 administering, 179, 180
Vertigo, 198, 199
Viral infections, 291

Wandering pacemaker, 1–2
 ectopic firing distinguished from,
 1
Wellens, H., 27
Wenckebach block, 87, 90–92, 97, 98,
 114, 117, 118, 120, 122, 158, 160,
 336, 357
 antegrade, 337
 bundle-branch, 188, 183–190
 exit, 189, 341
 intra-Hisian, 122
 in presence of atrial flutter,
 147–148
 retrograde, 332, 337
 reverse phenomenon, 337
 typical and atypical, 91
Wide-beat tachycardia, 17–31,
 178–182, 327, 329, 333
 during atrial fibrillation, 64
 basic skills for recognizing, 17
 bundle-branch block, 18–21
 capture beats, 25–29
 diagnosis of, 344
 differential diagnosis of, 17–31
 dissociation, 21–23
 fusion beats, 23–24, 25, 26
 junctional, 17, 30–31
 prognosis and treatment of, 17,
 29
 ventricular, 17, 27, 30
Wolff-Parkinson-White (WPW) preexcitation, 36, 162–164, 165, 167,
 319, 331
 Type A, 163, 171
 Type B, 164